International Ophthalmology Clinics

International Ophthalmology Clinics (ISSN 0020-8167) (ISBN 0-316-31916-3). Published quarterly by Little, Brown and Company, 34 Beacon Street, Boston, Massachusetts 02108-1493. Send address changes and subscription orders to Little, Brown and Company, Subscription Department, PO Box 2033, Langhorne, PA 19047-9480; (800) 628-4221. Subscription rates per year: personal subscription, U.S. and possessions, $81; foreign (includes Mexico), $105; Canada, $92; institutional, U.S., $99; foreign, $129; Canada, $109. Special rates for students, interns and residents per year: U.S., $55; foreign, $75; Canada, $65. Single copies: $30 for subscribers, $38 for nonsubscribers. In Japan please contact our exclusive agent: Medsi, 1-2-13 Yushima, Bunkyo-ku, Tokyo 113, Japan. Subscription rates per year in Japan: individual, ¥22,200; institutional, ¥26,200 (air cargo service only). Second-class postage paid at Boston, Massachusetts, and at additional mailing offices.

Postmaster: Send address changes to International Ophthalmology Clinics, PO Box 2033, Langhorne, PA 19047-9480.

International Ophthalmology Clinics is indexed in Index Medicus, Current Contents/Clinical Practice, Excerpta Medica, and Current Awareness in Biological Sciences.

International Ophthalmology Clinics

Volume 31
Number 3
Summer 1991

Systemic Associations of Ocular Disorders

EDITED BY

Daniel H. Gold, M.D.

*University of Texas Medical Branch
and Eye Clinic of Texas, Galveston, Texas*

Little, Brown and Company
BOSTON

Editors

Gilbert Smolin, M.D.
F.I. Proctor Foundation, San Francisco
Department of Ophthalmology,
University of California, San Francisco
Medical Center

Mitchell H. Friedlaender, M.D.
Division of Ophthalmology,
Scripps Clinic and Research Foundation,
La Jolla, California

Editorial Office
931 West San Bruno Avenue
San Bruno, CA 94066

Publisher
Little, Brown and Company, Boston, Massachusetts

Publishing Staff

Publisher
Lynne Herndon

Executive Editor
Christine F. Lamb

Managing Editor
Sherri Frank

Sales and Marketing Manager
Anne Orens

Production Manager
Fredda Purgalin

Editorial Board

Contents

Contributing Authors

Daniel H. Gold, M.D., EDITOR
University of Texas Medical Branch and
Eye Clinic of Texas
Galveston, TX
Address correspondence to:
2302 Avenue P
Galveston, TX 77550

Robert C. Arffa, M.D.
The Eye and Ear Institute
Pittsburgh, PA
Address correspondence to:
Allegheny General Hospital
420 East North Avenue
Pittsburgh, PA 15212

Gary C. Brown, M.D.
Retinovitreous Associates, Ltd.
910 E. Willow Grove Avenue
Philadelphia, PA 19118

Arlene V. Drack, M.D.
The Wilmer Ophthalmological Institute
The Johns Hopkins Hospital
600 N. Wolfe Street
Maumenee 321
Baltimore, MD 21205

Michael J. Elman, M.D.
University of Maryland
School of Medicine, *and*
Retina Service
Franklin Square Hospital
Baltimore, MD
Address correspondence to:
University of Maryland Professional Building
419 W. Redwood Street, Suite 460
Baltimore, MD 21201

F. Rodney Eve, M.D., F.R.C.S.
University of Texas Medical Branch
Galveston, TX
Address correspondence to:
807 Craig Street
Corpus Christi, TX 78404

Elizabeth M. Graham, M.R.C.P.
The Medical Eye Unit
St. Thomas' Hospital
Lambeth Palace Road
London SE1 7EH
England

Kim N. Hakin, F.R.C.S., F.C.Ophth.
Moorfields Eye Hospital
London EC1V 2PD
England

Ian Kaden, M.D.
Department of Ophthalmology
Montefiore Medical Center—University Hospital
Albert Einstein College of Medicine
Bronx, NY 10467

Ahmad M. Mansour, M.D.
Department of Ophthalmology
University of Texas Medical Branch
Galveston, TX 77550

Hector M. Marines, M.D.
Ophthalmic Plastic and Orbital Surgery
Cullen Eye Institute
Baylor College of Medicine
6501 Fannin, NC200
Houston, TX 77030

Martin Mayers, M.D.
Department of Ophthalmology
Montefiore Medical Center—University Hospital
Albert Einstein College of Medicine
Bronx, NY 10467

John A. McCrary, III, M.D.
Department of Ophthalmology
Cullen Eye Institute
Baylor College of Medicine
6501 Fannin, NC200
Houston, TX 77030

James R. Patrinely, M.D.
Department of Ophthalmology
Division of Plastic Surgery
Cullen Eye Institute
Baylor College of Medicine
6501 Fannin, NC200
Houston, TX 77030

James T. Rosenbaum, M.D.
Departments of Medicine, Ophthalmology, and Cell Biology
Oregon Health Sciences University
3181 S.W. Sam Jackson Park Road L329A
Portland, OR 97201

Miles R. Stanford, F.R.C.S.
The Medical Eye Unit
St. Thomas' Hospital
Lambeth Palace Road
London SE1 7EH
England

Elias I. Traboulsi, M.D.
The Wilmer Ophthalmological Institute
The Johns Hopkins Hospital
600 N. Wolfe Street
Maumenee 321
Baltimore, MD 21205

Peter G. Watson, F.R.C.S., F.C.Ophth.
Moorfields Eye Hospital
London EC1V 2PD
England

Preface

No medical problem can be properly understood as an isolated entity but must be seen in relation to the larger picture of a patient's general health and life patterns. Despite the obvious truth of this traditional medical maxim, it is often overlooked when the pressing needs of acute events force us to focus on problems that require more immediate attention.

The spectrum of ocular problems with significant systemic associations is extensive. These involve almost every ocular structure, from the cornea and sclera externally to the uvea and retina internally, from the lacrimal system anteriorly to the optic nerve and orbit posteriorly.

A volume such as this cannot hope to cover such a broad range of material in any comprehensive way or even to review briefly all the ocular–systemic associations that have been discovered over the years. The aim of this issue of *International Ophthalmology Clinics* is to raise our level of awareness of these interrelationships and to stimulate a search for them in our patients, a search that will inevitably benefit both our patients and ourselves.

Daniel H. Gold

Systemic Associations of Retinal Arterial Obstructive Disease

Gary C. Brown, M.D.

Arterial obstructive disease can affect the posterior segment of the eye in a number of ways. Carotid artery obstruction can lead to the ocular ischemic syndrome, whereas central retinal artery and branch retinal artery obstructions generally cause retinal whitening and acute visual loss. Blockage of retinal arterioles can manifest in the form of cotton-wool spots. Despite their differing clinical appearances, these entities share certain common, underlying systemic diseases. This chapter describes the various arterial obstructive phenomena that can affect the eye, from the larger vessels down to the smaller vessels, including ophthalmoscopic findings and systemic associations.

■ Ocular Ischemic Syndrome

Ocular ischemic syndrome is a term used to describe the ocular symptoms and signs occurring secondary to severe carotid artery obstruction [1]. Names used to designate the entity in the past have included *venous stasis retinopathy* [2], *ischemic ocular inflammation* [3], and *ischemic oculopathy* [4].

Symptoms of the ocular ischemic syndrome include decreased vision in 90% of affected eyes and ocular or periocular pain in 40% [1]. Enlarged collateral vessels on the scalp are occasionally noted. Neovascularization of the iris (rubeosis iridis) is seen in approximately two-thirds of eyes.

Posterior segment findings include narrowed retinal arteries and dilated, but not tortuous, retinal veins in most eyes (Fig 1) [1]. Retinal hemorrhages (Fig 2) are found in 80% of eyes and neovascularization of the optic disc or retina can be seen in approximately 33%. Less frequently encountered signs include macular edema, a cherry-red spot, spontaneous retinal arterial pulsations, cotton-wool spots, and retinal arterial emboli. The optic disc is usually normal in appearance.

Intravenous fluorescein angiography reveals delayed choroidal filling in 60% of eyes, an increased retinal arteriovenous transit time in 95%, and late staining of the larger retinal vessels (particularly the arteries) in 85% of eyes [1]. Macular edema, microaneurysms, and areas of retinal capillary nonperfusion are also frequently encountered.

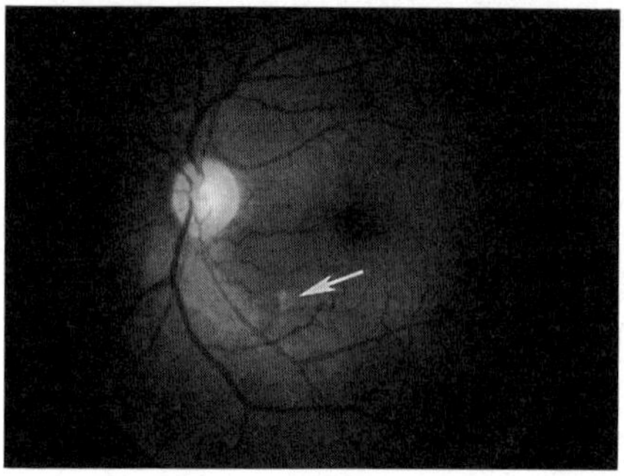

Figure 1 *Dilated retinal veins and narrowed retinal arteries in left eye of a woman with ocular ischemic syndrome. A cotton-wool spot* (arrow) *can be seen inferotemporal to the optic disc, and several small retinal hemorrhages are present.*

Typically, a 90% or greater stenosis of the ipsilateral internal or common carotid artery is necessary to cause the ocular ischemic syndrome. Obstruction of the innominate artery (aortic arch syndrome) [5] and chronic obstruction of the ophthalmic artery [6] are also occasionally responsible for the syndrome. Rarely, obstruction of the central retinal artery alone can cause it [7]. The predominant underlying etiology is atherosclerosis. Other possible causes, although unusual, include giant-cell arteritis, dissecting aneurysm, syphilitic arteritis, and Takayasu's disease [8].

Predictably, the ocular ischemic syndrome is frequently encountered in conjunction with entities associated with atherosclerosis. A list of these appears in Table 1 [9]. Systemic arterial hypertension is found in approximately three-fourths of cases [9], as compared to approximately one-fourth of an age-matched group in the Framingham Study [10]. More than half of the people with the ocular ischemic syndrome have diabetes mellitus, as compared to approximately 6% in an age-matched group [9, 10]. Almost 50% of persons with the ocular ischemic syndrome have evidence of ischemic heart disease, manifested by a history of previous myocardial infarction, the presence of angina pectoris, or electrocardiographic changes. More than 25% of patients have had a previous cerebrovascular accident at the time of diagnosis of the ocular ischemic syndrome. Nearly 20% have already required a peripheral bypass operation for the sequelae of atherosclerotic obstruction.

When persons with the ocular ischemic syndrome who have undergone

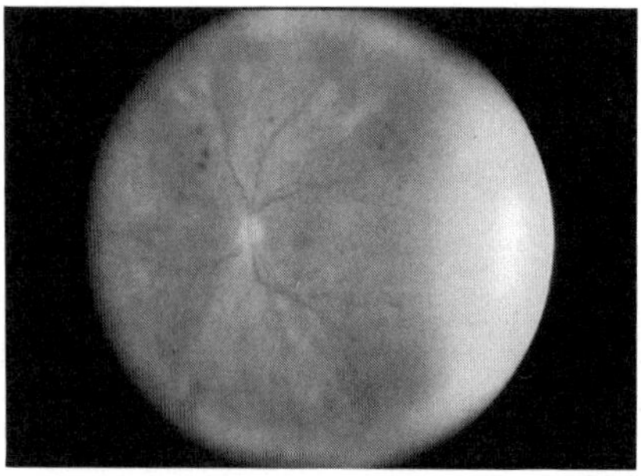

Figure 2 *Equator-plus photograph of left eye with ocular ischemic syndrome. Typical midperipheral dot and blot retinal hemorrhages are present.*

Table 1 *Systemic Diseases Associated with the Ocular Ischemic Syndrome [9]*

Disease	% of Patients
Systemic arterial hypertension	73
Diabetes mellitus	56
Ischemic heart disease	48
Cerebrovascular accident	27
Peripheral vascular disease	19

Source: Data from Sivalingam A et al, The ocular ischemic syndrome: II. Mortality and systemic morbidity. Int Ophthalmol 1989;13:187–191.

carotid endarterectomy or superficial temporal arterial to middle cerebral arterial bypass are included with those who have not undergone such surgery, the subsequent stroke rate is approximately 4% annually [9]. Age-matched data from the Framingham Study [10] reveal a comparable figure of 0.49% annually in those without the ocular ischemic syndrome. For reference, the yearly stroke rate in people with previous transient ischemic attack is approximately 8% [11]. Despite the increased stroke rate, cerebrovascular accident is not the leading cause of death in people with the ocular ischemic syndrome.

The 5-year mortality in persons with the ocular ischemic syndrome is nearly 40% (Fig 3) [9]. Cardiovascular disease is the leading cause of death, accounting for more than 60% of cases. Stroke is the cause of death in approximately 20%. Although the disease can present with ocular findings alone, the clinician should be aware that cardiac evaluation should not be neglected.

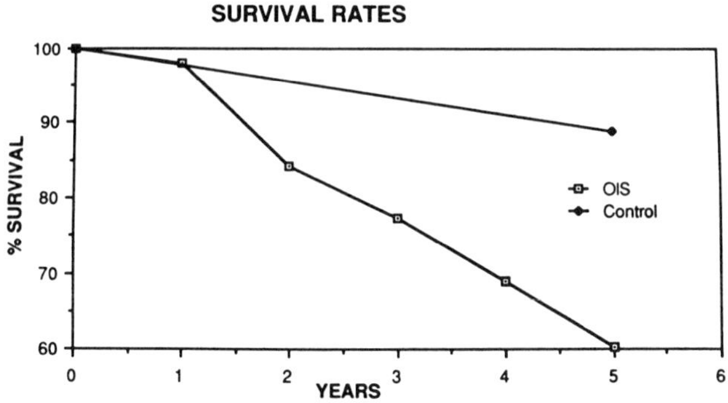

Figure 3 *Survival rate in persons with ocular ischemic syndrome (OIS) as compared to an age-matched group from the Framingham Study [10] without OIS. (From Sivalingam A et al, The ocular ischemic syndrome: II. Mortality and systemic morbidity. Int Ophthalmol 1989; 13:187–191.)*

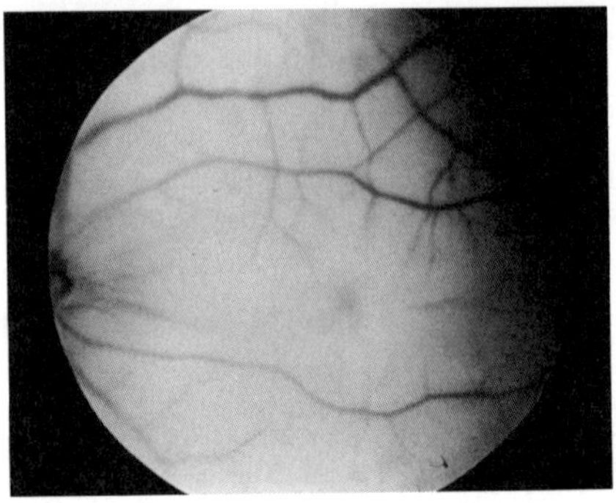

Figure 4 *Left fundus of 14-year-old child with acute ophthalmic artery obstruction from a knife injury. Marked retinal whitening is present and a cherry-red spot is absent. Visual acuity was no light perception. (Reprinted with permission from Brown GC, Magargal LE. Sudden occlusion of the retinal and posterior choroidal circulations in a youth. Am J Ophthalmol 1979;88:690–693. Copyright © Ophthalmic Publishing Company.)*

■ Ophthalmic Artery Obstruction

An acute ophthalmic artery obstruction appears clinically similar to a central retinal artery obstruction. There is a history of acute visual loss, an afferent pupillary defect is present, and superficial whitening of the retina is seen in the posterior pole [12]. In contrast to acute central retinal artery obstruction alone, acute ophthalmic artery obstruction is often associated with visual acuity of no light perception, more severe retinal whitening, and absence of a cherry-red spot (Fig 4). Late retinal pigment epithelial changes frequently arise owing to concomitant choroidal ischemia.

The systemic diseases associated with acute ophthalmic artery obstruction are similar to those found with acute central retinal artery obstruction, although substantially less information is available concerning the former condition. Two notable exceptions bear mentioning. Giant-cell arteritis can cause an acute ophthalmic artery obstruction. Thus, an erythrocyte sedimentation rate should probably be obtained in all affected persons older than 55 years unless another cause is present. Mucormycosis of the orbit is also a cause. The obstruction occurs secondary to a vasculitis induced by the organism [13]. Embolic etiologies should be investigated as well, particularly since the ophthalmic artery makes a right or acute angle in 40% of patients [14], an anatomical variant that could theoretically lead to the entrapment of emboli.

■ Central Retinal Artery Obstruction

Acute central retinal artery obstruction usually causes severe visual loss, most commonly to the range of counting fingers to hand motions. Characteristic fundus appearance includes narrowed retinal arteries, superficial retinal whitening in the posterior pole, and a cherry-red spot in the foveola (Fig 5).

Pathophysiological Mechanisms

A number of basic pathophysiological mechanisms have been shown to cause central retinal artery obstruction, including emboli [15, 16], intraluminal thrombosis [17], hemorrhage under atherosclerotic plaque [17, 18], spasm [19–21], vasculitis [16, 22], dissecting aneurysm [23], hypertensive arteriolar

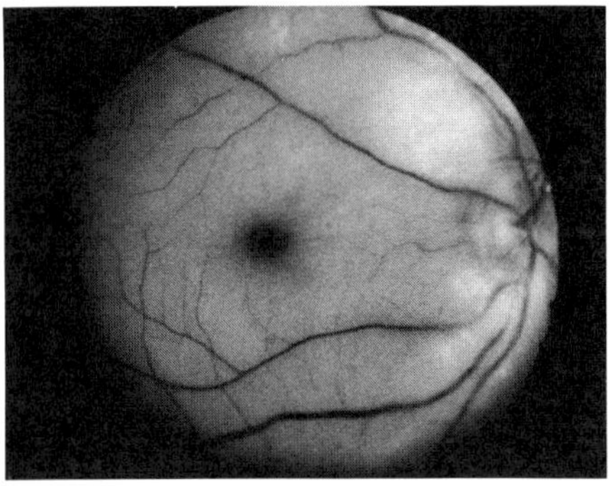

Figure 5 *Fundus of an eye with acute central retinal artery obstruction. Superficial retinal whitening is present, as is a cherry-red spot in the foveola.*

necrosis [24], and circulatory collapse [25]. For the most part, the processes responsible for acute central retinal artery obstruction and branch retinal artery obstruction are similar.

Associated Diseases

Numerous specific disease entities have been associated with retinal artery obstruction [12, 13, 15, 16, 19–21, 45–70]. Many are listed in Table 2. It must be noted, however, that the list may not be complete.

Arterial Hypertension Systemic arterial hypertension is present in approximately two-thirds of people with central retinal artery obstruction [15]. Possible mechanisms by which it can contribute to central retinal artery obstruction include enhancement of atherosclerotic plaque formation, spasm, vascular necrosis, and hemorrhage under an atherosclerotic plaque [18–24]. The mean age of persons with central retinal artery obstruction is in the sixties, the same as those with the ocular ischemic syndrome [1, 15]. The incidence of systemic arterial hypertension in an uninvolved age-matched group is approximately 25% [10].

Diabetes Mellitus Diabetes mellitus is encountered in nearly one-fourth of people with central retinal artery obstruction [15]. The incidence for an age-matched group would be expected to be in the 6 to 7% range [10].

Carotid Atherosclerosis and Cardiac Valvular Disease The two most common entities responsible for embolic central retinal artery obstruction are atherosclerotic carotid artery disease and cardiac valvular disease [15, 16]. Intraarterial retinal emboli are found in approximately 20% of eyes with acute central retinal artery obstruction [15]. Carotid atherosclerosis [27], as defined by an ipsilateral stenosis or a plaque seen with digital subtraction angiography, is present in 45% or so of cases. In about 20% of people, the atherosclerosis causes a 50% or greater stenosis. Typically, emboli from carotid atherosclerotic disease manifest as glistening, yellow or golden, intraarterial foci (Hollenhorst plaques [Fig 6]). They are often multiple and, due to their small size, may not cause obstruction. In some eyes with central retinal artery obstruction, a pale yellow embolus is seen on the optic disc in conjunction with small cholesterol emboli elsewhere in the fundus. It is likely, in these instances,

Table 2 *Systemic and Ocular Abnormalities That Have Been Associated with Retinal Artery Obstruction*

Entities contributing to embolus formation
Arterial hypertension (via atherosclerotic plaque formation) [15, 25]
Carotid atherosclerosis [16, 26–28]
Cardiac valvular disease
  Rheumatic [15, 16, 25]
  Mitral valve prolapse [29, 30]
Mural thrombus after myocardial infarction [31]
Atrial myxoma [32, 33]
Tumors [34]
Intravenous drug abuse [35, 36]
Lipid emboli
  Pancreatitis [37]
  Purtscher's retinopathy (trauma) [38]
Loiasis [39, 40]
Radiological studies
  Carotid angiography [41]
  Lymphangiography [42]
  Hysterosalpingography [43]
  Ventriculography [44]
Head and neck corticosteroid injection [45]
Retrobulbar corticosteroids [46]

Trauma (via compression, spasm, or direct vessel damage)
Retrobulbar injection [47–49]
Orbital fracture repair [36, 50, 51]
General anesthesia [52]
Penetrating injury [53]
Drug- or alcohol-induced stupor [12]

Coagulopathies
Sickle cell disease [36, 54, 55]
Homocystinuria [56]
Oral contraceptives [36, 57]
Platelet and factor abnormalities [36]
Pregnancy [36]
Lupus anticoagulants [58]
Protein S deficiency [59]

Ocular conditions associated with retinal artery obstruction
Prepapillary arterial loops [60, 61]
Optic disc drusen [36, 62]
Increased intraocular pressure (with sickling hemoglobinopathy) [36, 54]

Collagen vascular diseases
Systemic lupus erythematosus [36, 63, 64]
Polyarteritis nodosa [25]
Giant-cell arteritis [65]

Other associations
Fabry's disease [66]
Sydenham's chorea [67]
Migraine [19–21, 36]
Hypotension [25]
Fibromuscular hyperplasia [68]
Optic neuritis [69]
Orbital mucormycosis [12, 13]
Radiation retinopathy [70]

Source: Modified from Brown GC, Retinal arterial obstructive disease. In: Ryan JJ, ed. Retina, vol 2. St Louis: Mosby, 1989:403–419.

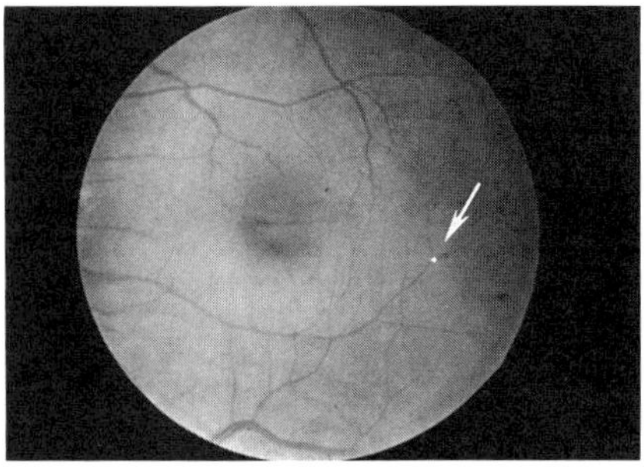

Figure 6 *Glistening yellow cholesterol embolus* (arrow) *at a bifurcation within retinal arterial system. Also known as Hollenhorst plaques, they are believed to originate from carotid arteries.*

that the embolus on the disc is also a cholesterol embolus but appears different because it is surrounded by a fibrin-platelet thrombus.

Emboli of cardiac origin can occur secondary to rheumatic heart disease [15, 16, 25], mitral valve prolapse [29, 30], mural thrombi after myocardial infarction [31], or myxomas [32, 33]. The calcific emboli from rheumatic valvular disease tend to be larger and whiter in appearance than their cholesterol counterparts (Fig 7). Because of their greater size, they have an increased tendency to cause clinically apparent arterial obstruction.

The observation of a retinal artery embolus, whether associated or unassociated with retinal artery obstruction, suggests poor long-term survival. Savino and associates [71] found a 9-year survival rate of 44% in persons with retinal arterial emboli, as compared to 73% in an age-matched and sex-matched group without emboli.

Collagen Vascular Disorders Giant-cell arteritis can cause central retinal artery obstruction but probably only accounts for 1 to 2% of cases [68]. Theoretically, it can also cause blockage of the larger retinal branch arteries, although the incidence of the occurrence is unknown. An erythrocyte sedimentation rate to screen for this entity should be undertaken in older people with no readily apparent cause for a retinal artery obstruction. Other collagen vascular

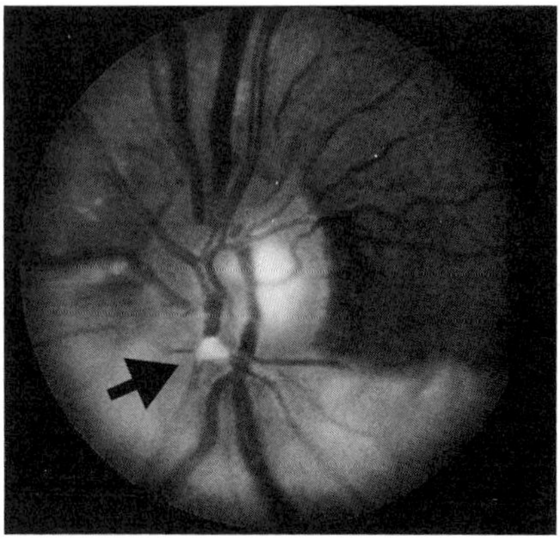

Figure 7 *White calcific plaque* (arrow) *causing obstruction within the inferior papillary retinal artery. Calcific emboli tend to be larger than the cholesterol variant and, more frequently than not, cause arterial obstruction when entrapped in retinal arteries. These emboli are believed to usually arise from the aortic valve.*

diseases that have been associated with central retinal artery obstruction include polyarteritis nodosa [25] and systemic lupus erythematosus [36, 63, 64].

Trauma Surgical and external trauma can lead to retinal artery obstruction [47–53]. Possible mechanisms after retrobulbar injection for ocular surgery include direct damage to the central retinal artery from the needle, spasm, and hemorrhage within the optic nerve sheath causing compression. Combined obstructions of the central retinal artery and central retinal vein are a variant of retinal artery obstruction that has been reported after retrobulbar injection [49, 68]. Extended pressure on the globe when the patient is in a supine position for neurosurgical procedures can also lead to central retinal artery obstruction, usually with concomitant shutdown of the choroidal circulation [12, 52].

Coagulopathies Coagulopathies have been associated with central retinal artery obstruction. Sickling hemoglobinopathies are a cause, including sickle cell trait, when the intraocular pressure is rapidly raised above normal [36, 54, 55]. This is particularly pertinent in cases of traumatic hyphema leading to secondary glaucoma. Aggressive management to lower an elevated intraocular pressure should be considered in these instances. Another abnormality in this group is the presence of antiphospholipid antibodies (lupus anticoagulants) [58]. Persons with lupus anticoagulants (antibodies of the IgM or IgG class with an affinity for anionic phospholipids) often have a prolonged partial thromboplastin time. Multisystem thromboses of both the arteries and veins commonly occur in affected people.

Local Ocular Abnormalities Local ocular abnormalities can contribute to retinal artery obstruction. Prepapillary arterial loops are believed to predispose to turbulence of retinal blood flow, with subsequent endothelial cell damage and thrombus formation [60, 61]. Optic nerve drusen are believed to compress the central retinal artery in the prelaminar region of the nerve head, again predisposing to turbulence and thrombus formation [62]. Increased intraocular pressure can predispose persons with sickling hemoglobinopathy to central retinal artery obstruction, as it can in those with the ocular ischemic syndrome. In this latter instance, it has been proposed that neovascular glaucoma leads to an increased intraocular pressure that compromises central retinal artery flow [1, 72].

Age-Related Differences In children and adults younger than 30 years, the causes of retinal artery obstruction are often different from those in the older population [36]. Carotid atherosclerosis is a most unusual cause in this age group. Abnormalities more frequently encountered in younger people with retinal artery obstruction include migraine, coagulation abnormalities, cardiac disorders, trauma, sickling hemoglobinopathies, and local abnormalities, such as prepapillary arterial loops and optic nerve drusen.

Diagnostic Workup

A systemic history and physical examination in conjunction with a thorough fundus examination often provide information concerning the cause

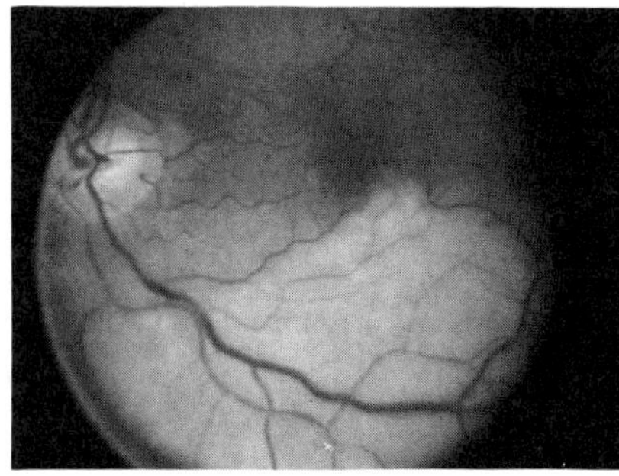

Figure 8 *Segmental, superficial retinal whitening typical of branch retinal artery obstruction.*

of retinal artery obstruction. A laboratory workup is generally undertaken, depending on the physical findings and individual patient.

■ Branch Retinal Artery Obstruction

The causes of branch retinal artery obstruction (Fig 8) are similar to those of central retinal artery obstruction, with minor differences. Since the branch retinal arteries lose the internal elastic lamina and have a marked diminution of the media in the vessel wall within several millimeters after entering from the optic disc, atherosclerosis does not form peripherally in these vessels [73]. Rather than arteries, the vessels become arterioles. Thus, hemorrhage under an atherosclerotic plaque, or associated thrombus formation due to an ulcerated plaque, is a less likely mechanism for obstruction with branch retinal arteries than with the central retinal artery. Giant-cell arteritis is also believed not to involve the more distal retinal arterioles.

Emboli have a tendency to be trapped at arterial bifurcations in the retina owing to narrowing of the lumina distal to the point of division. Thus, branch retinal artery obstructions are more likely to have an embolic etiology when they arise at points of bifurcation. Those occurring at other sites are less likely to have an embolic cause.

■ Cilioretinal Artery Obstruction

A cilioretinal artery is a vessel that generally arises on the more peripheral aspect of the optic disc, separate from the central retinal artery. These vessels have been shown to originate from the short posterior ciliary arteries and the choroidal circulation [74]. The causes of cilioretinal artery obstruction are similar to those of central retinal artery obstruction [75].

Cilioretinal artery obstruction can occur as an isolated entity or in conjunction with central retinal vein obstruction or anterior ischemic optic neuropathy [75]. With instances of central retinal vein obstruction and concomitant cilioretinal artery obstruction, it has been suggested that swelling of the surrounding optic nerve can compromise blood flow through the cilioretinal artery and lead to thrombus formation (Fig 9) [75]. These cases frequently are noted in a younger age group than those with other forms of arterial obstructive disease of the retina [75, 76]. Often, no underlying systemic cause is found. Cilioretinal

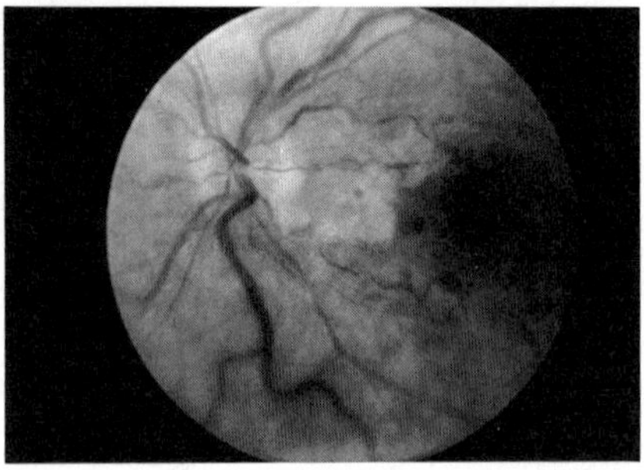

Figure 9 *Mild central retinal vein obstruction associated with cilioretinal artery obstruction in left eye of a 26-year-old woman. Systemic workup was normal.*

artery obstruction in conjunction with anterior ischemic optic neuropathy usually occurs in an elderly population. The possibility of the presence of giant-cell arteritis should be considered in this latter situation.

■ Cotton-Wool Spots

Cotton-wool spots, or soft exudates, appear ophthalmoscopically as small, yellow-white, superficial retinal lesions that generally occupy an area less than one-fourth that of the optic disc (see Fig 1). The abnormalities usually do not cause central visual loss and often disappear within 5 to 7 weeks [77]. They can occur singly, but most commonly are multiple and are seen in conjunction with other fundus abnormalities, such as retinal hemorrhages, microaneurysms, and hard exudates. Confined to the posterior aspect of the retina, they correlate with areas of focal retinal ischemia that cause axoplasmic blockage [78].

The most common cause of cotton-wool spots is diabetic retinopathy. In the presence of a normal fasting glucose level, a glucose tolerance test may be necessary to rule out the possibility of latent diabetes mellitus [79]. In general, retinal microaneurysms and hemorrhages accompany cotton-wool spots in eyes with diabetic retinopathy.

Entities known to be associated with cotton-wool spots are listed in Table 3, although other associations probably exist. Additionally, most abnormalities that cause central or branch retinal artery obstruction can also produce cotton-wool spots. After diabetes, the disease entities most frequently seen in conjunction with cotton-wool spots are retinal venous obstruction, systemic arterial hypertension, collagen vascular diseases, and the acquired immunodeficiency syndrome (AIDS) [79].

The diastolic blood pressure generally is 110 mm Hg or greater in persons who have cotton-wool spots secondary to systemic arterial hypertension [80]. Since cotton-wool spots usually resolve within several weeks after their appearance, the presence of these abnormalities indicates recent poor blood pressure control. Fibrinoid necrosis may be the mechanism that causes the arteriolar obstruction producing localized ischemia and axoplasmic blocking in the eyes of extremely hypertensive individuals [81].

A cause of cotton-wool spots that is being seen with increased frequency is AIDS [82]. Cotton-wool spots have been reported ophthalmoscopically in 27 to 53% of eyes in AIDS patients. Infectious organisms have not been isolated

Table 3 *Abnormalities Associated with the Presence of Cotton-Wool Spots in the Fundus*

Diabetes mellitus
Systemic arterial hypertension
Collagen vascular disease
Systemic lupus erythematosus
Dermatomyositis
Polyarteritis nodosa
Scleroderma
Giant-cell arteritis
Cardiac valvular disease
Mitral valve prolapse
Rheumatic heart disease
Endocarditis
Human immunodeficiency virus (HIV) infection
Leukemia
Trauma
Radiation retinopathy
Retinal venous obstruction
Metastatic carcinoma
Leptospirosis
Partial central retinal artery obstruction
Rocky Mountain spotted fever
High-altitude retinopathy
Severe anemia
Acute blood loss
Papilledema
Papillitis
Ocular ischemic syndrome (carotid artery atherosclerosis)
Dysproteinemias
Septicemia
Aortic arch syndromes
Intravenous drug abuse
Acute pancreatitis
Onchocerciasis
Lupus anticoagulant retinopathy

Source: Adapted from Brown GC et al, Cotton-wool spots. Retina 1985;5:206–214.

from the lesions. Their cause is unknown, but it has been proposed that a deposition of immune complexes within retinal arterioles may be responsible.

The importance of even a single cotton-wool spot in the fundus should not be underestimated. Excluding persons with known diabetes mellitus, Brown and associates [79] found a potentially serious underlying systemic disease in 95% of patients with a fundus appearance characterized by a predominance of cotton-wool spots or a single cotton-wool spot.

■ References

1. Brown GC, Magargal LE. The ocular ischemic syndrome. Clinical, fluorescein angiographic and carotid angiographic features. Int Ophthalmol 1988;11:239–251
2. Kearns TP, Hollenhorst RW. Venous-stasis retinopathy of occlusive disease of the carotid artery. Proc Mayo Clin 1963;38:304–312
3. Knox DL. Ischemic ocular inflammation. Am J Ophthalmol 1965;60:995–1002

4. Young LHY, Appen RE. Ischemic oculopathy. A manifestation of carotid artery disease. Arch Neurol 1981;38:358–361
5. Kearns TP. Ophthalmology and the carotid artery. Am J Ophthalmol 1979;88: 714–722
6. Madsen PH. Venous-stasis insufficiency of the ophthalmic artery. Acta Ophthalmol (Copenh) 1965;44:940–947
7. Magargal LE, Sanborn GE, Zimmermann A. Venous stasis retinopathy associated with embolic obstruction of the central retinal artery. J Clin Neuro Ophthalmol 1982;2:113–118
8. Chambers JK, Henkind P. Arterial occlusive disease of the retina. In: Duane TD, ed. Clinical ophthalmology, vol 3, chap 14. Hagerstown, MD: Harper & Row, 1983:1–14
9. Sivalingam A, Brown GC, Magargal LE, Menduke H. The ocular ischemic syndrome: II. Mortality and systemic morbidity. Int Ophthalmol 1989;13:187–191
10. Kannel WB, Gordon T, eds. The Framingham Study. Public Health Service Publication No. NIH 77-1247, 1977: section 6, tables 6–9; section 29, tables A-22 and A-23; section 32, pp 84–85
11. Easton JT, Hart RG, Sherman DG, Kaste M. Diagnosis and management of ischemic stroke (pt 1). Threatened stroke and its management. Curr Probl Cardiol 1983;8:76
12. Brown GC, Magargal LE, Sergott R. Acute obstruction of the retinal and choroidal circulations. Ophthalmology 1986;93:1373–1382
13. Gass JDM. Ocular manifestations of acute mucormycosis. Arch Ophthalmol 1961; 65:226–237
14. Hayreh SS, Dass R. The ophthalmic artery: II. Intra-orbital course. Br J Ophthalmol 1962;46:165–185
15. Brown GC, Magargal LE. Central retinal artery obstruction and visual acuity. Ophthalmology 1982;89:14–19
16. Appen RE, Wray SH, Cogan DG. Central retinal artery occlusion. Am J Ophthalmol 1975;79:374–381
17. Perraut LE, Zimmerman LE. The occurrence of glaucoma following occlusion of the central retinal artery. A clinicopathologic report of six cases with a review of the literature. Arch Ophthalmol 1959;61:845–865
18. Dahrling BE. The histopathology of early central retinal artery occlusion. Arch Ophthalmol 1965;73:506–510
19. Carroll D. Retinal migraine. Headache 1970;10:9–13
20. Graveson GS. Retinal arterial occlusion in migraine. Br Med J 1949;2:838–840
21. Silberberg DH, Laties AM. Occlusive migraine. Trans Pa Acad Ophthalmol Otolaryngol 1974;27:34–38
22. Karjalainen K. Occlusion of the central retinal artery and branch retinal arterioles. Acta Ophthalmol [Suppl] (Copenh) 1971;109:5–96
23. Wolter JR, Hansen KD. Intimo-intimal intussusception of the central retinal artery. Am J Ophthalmol 1981;92:486–491
24. Leishman R. The eye in general vascular disease. Hypertension and arteriosclerosis. Br J Ophthalmol 1957;41:641–701
25. Gold D. Retinal arterial occlusion. Trans Am Acad Ophthalmol Otolaryngol 1977;83:392–408
26. Savino PJ, Glaser JS, Cassady J. Retinal stroke. Is the patient at risk? Arch Ophthalmol 1977;95:1185–1189
27. Shah HG, Brown GC, Goldberg RE. Digital subtraction carotid angiography and retinal arterial obstruction. Ophthalmology 1985;92:68–72
28. Kollarits CR, Lubow M, Hissong SL. Retinal strokes: I. Incidence of carotid atheromata. JAMA 1972;222:1273–1275
29. Woldoff HS, Gerber M, Desser KB, Benchimol A. Retinal vascular lesions in two patients with prolapsed mitral valve leaflets. Am J Ophthalmol 1975;79:382–385

30. Wilson LA, Keeling PWN, Malcolm AD, et al. Visual complications of mitral leaf prolapse. Br Med J 1977;2:86–88
31. Zimmerman LE. Embolism of central retinal artery secondary to myocardial infarction with mural thrombosis. Arch Ophthalmol 1975;73:822–826
32. Jampol LM, Wong AS, Albert DM. Atrial myxoma and central retinal artery occlusion. Am J Ophthalmol 1973;75:242–249
33. Cogan DG, Wray SH. Vascular occlusions in the eye from cardiac myxomas. Am J Ophthalmol 1975;80:396–403
34. Tarkkanen A, Merenmies L, Makinen J. Embolism of central retinal artery secondary to metastatic carcinoma. Acta Ophthalmol (Copenh) 1973;51:25–33
35. Atlee WE. Talc and cornstarch emboli in eyes of drug abusers. JAMA 1972;219:49–51
36. Brown GC, Magargal LE, Shields JA, et al. Retinal arterial obstruction in children and young adults. Ophthalmology 1981;88:18–25
37. Inkeles DM, Walsh JB. Retinal fat emboli as a sequela to acute pancreatitis. Am J Ophthalmol 1975;80:935–938
38. Madsen PH. Traumatic retinal angiopathy (Purtscher). Ophthalmologica 1972;165:453–458
39. Toussaint D, Danis P. Retinopathy in generalized Loa-loa filariasis. A clinicopathological study. Arch Ophthalmol 1965;74:470–476
40. Corrigan MJ, Hill DW. Retinal arterial occlusion in loiasis. Br J Ophthalmol 1968;52:477–480
41. Carlson MR, Pilger IS, Rosenbaum AL. Central retinal artery occlusion after carotid angiography. Am J Ophthalmol 1976;81:103–104
42. Rasmussen KE. Retinal and cerebral fat emboli following lymphography with oily contrast media. Acta Radiol 1970;10:199–202
43. Charawanamutta AM, Hughes-Nurse J, Hamlett JD. Retinal embolism after hysterosalpingography. Br J Ophthalmol 1973;57:166–169
44. Keane JR. Sudden blindness after ventriculography. Bilateral retinal vascular occlusion superimposed on papilledema. Am J Ophthalmol 1974;78:275–278
45. Wilson RS, Havener WH, McGrew RN. Bilateral retinal artery and choriocapillaris occlusion following the injection of long-acting corticosteroid suspensions in combination with other drugs: I. Clinical studies. Ophthalmology 1978;85:967–974
46. Ellis PP. Occlusion of the central retinal artery after retrobulbar corticosteroid injection. Am J Ophthalmol 1978;85:352–356
47. Klein ML, Jampol LM, Condon PI, et al. Central retinal artery occlusion without retrobulbar hemorrhage after retrobulbar anesthesia. Am J Ophthalmol 1982;93:573–577
48. Kraushar MF, Seelenfreund MH, Freilich DB. Central retinal artery closure during orbital hemorrhage from retrobulbar injection. Trans Am Acad Ophthalmol Otolaryngol 1974;78:65–70
49. Sullivan K, Brown GC, Forman AR, et al. Retrobulbar anesthesia and retinal vascular obstruction. Ophthalmology 1983;90:373–377
50. Emery JM, Huff JD, Justice J. Central retinal artery occlusion after blowout fracture repair. Am J Ophthalmol 1974;78:538–540
51. Nicholson DH, Guzak SV. Visual loss complicating repair of orbital floor fractures. Arch Ophthalmol 1971;86:369–375
52. Hollenhorst RW, Svien HJ, Benoit CF. Unilateral blindness occurring during anesthesia for neurosurgical operations. Arch Ophthalmol 1954;52:819–830
53. Brown GC, Magargal LE. Sudden occlusion of the retinal and posterior choroidal circulations in a youth. Am J Ophthalmol 1979;88:690–693
54. Michelson PE, Pfaffenbach D. Retinal arterial occlusion following ocular trauma in youths with sickle-trait hemoglobinopathy. Am J Ophthalmol 1972;74:494–497

55. Sorr EM, Goldberg RE. Traumatic central retinal artery occlusion with sickle cell trait. Am J Ophthalmol 1975;80:648–652
56. Wilson RS, Ruiz RS. Bilateral central retinal artery occlusion in homocystinuria. A case report. Arch Ophthalmol 1969;82:267–268
57. Friedman S, Golan A, Schoenfeld A, Goldman J. Acute ophthalmologic complications during the use of oral contraceptives. Contraception 1974;10:685–692
58. Kleiner RC, Najarian LV, Schatten S, et al. Vaso-occlusive retinopathy associated with anti-phospholipid antibodies (lupus anticoagulant retinopathy). Ophthalmology 1989;96:896–904
59. Greven CM, Weaver RG, Owen J, Slusher MM. Protein S deficiency and bilateral branch retinal artery occlusion. Ophthalmology 1991;98:33–34
60. Brown GC, Magargal LE, Augsburger JA, Shields JA. Preretinal arterial loops and retinal arterial occlusion. Am J Ophthalmol 1979;87:646–651
61. Degenhart W, Brown GC, Augsburger JJ, Magargal LE. Prepapillary vascular loops. Ophthalmology 1981;88:1126–1131
62. Purcell JJ, Goldberg RE. Hyaline bodies of the optic papilla and bilateral acute vascular occlusions. Ann Ophthalmol 1974;6:1069–1076
63. Gold DH, Morris DA, Henkind P. Ocular findings in systemic lupus erythematosus. Br J Ophthalmol 1972;56:800–804
64. Wong K, Ai E, Jones JV, Young D. Visual loss as the initial symptom of systemic lupus erythematosus. Am J Ophthalmol 1981;92:238–244
65. Eagling EM, Sanders MD, Miller JJH. Ischemic papillopathy. Clinical and fluorescein angiographic review of forty cases. Br J Ophthalmol 1974;58:990–1008
66. Sher NA, Reiff W, Letson RD, Desnick RJ. Central retinal artery occlusion complicating Fabry's disease. Arch Ophthalmol 1978;96:815–817
67. Ling W, Oftedal G, Simon T. Central retinal artery occlusion in Sydenham's chorea. Am J Dis Child 1969;118:525–527
68. Brown GC. Retinal arterial obstructive disease. In: Ryan SJ, ed. Retina, vol 2. St Louis: Mosby, 1989:403–419
69. Brown GC, Tasman WS. Retinal arterial obstruction in association with presumed *Toxocara canis* neuroretinitis. Ann Ophthalmol 1981;13:1385–1387
70. Brown GC, Shields JA, Sanborn G, et al. Radiation retinopathy. Ophthalmology 1982;89:1494–1501
71. Savino PJ, Glaser JS, Cassady J. Retinal stroke. Is the patient at risk? Arch Ophthalmol 1977;95:1185–1189
72. Brown GC, Magargal LE, Simeone FE, et al. Arterial obstruction and ocular neovascularization. Ophthalmology 1982;89:139–146
73. Brownstein S, Font RL, Alper M. Atheromatous plaques in the retinal blood vessels. Arch Ophthalmol 1973;90:49–52
74. Hayreh SS. The cilio-retinal arteries. Br J Ophthalmol 1963;47:71–89
75. Brown GC, Moffat K, Cruess A, et al. Cilioretinal artery obstruction. Retina 1983;3:182–187
76. McLeon D, Ring CP. Cilio-retinal infarction after retinal vein occlusion. Br J Ophthalmol 1976;60:419–427
77. Kohner EM, Dollery CT, Bulpitt CJ. Cotton-wool spots in diabetic retinopathy. Diabetes 1969;18:691–704
78. McLeod D, Marshall J, Kohner EM, Bird AC. The role of axoplasmic transport in the pathogenesis of retinal cotton-wool spots. Br J Ophthalmol 1977;61:177–191
79. Brown GC, Brown MM, Hiller T, et al. Cotton-wool spots. Retina 1985;5:206–214
80. Brown GC, Benson WE. The fundus manifestations of malignant hypertension. Trans Pa Acad Ophthalmol Otolaryngol 1984;37:19–25
81. Garner A, Ashton N, Tripathi R, et al. Pathogenesis of hypertensive retinopathy. Br J Ophthalmol 1975;59:3–44
82. Freeman WR, Helm M. Retinal and ophthalmologic manifestations of AIDS. In: Ryan SJ, ed. Retina, vol 2. St Louis: Mosby, 1989:597–615

Systemic Associations of Retinal Vein Occlusion

Michael J. Elman, M.D.

Retinal vein occlusion may result in profound and permanent visual loss [1–6]. Central retinal vein occlusion (CRVO) results from thrombosis of the central retinal vein [7]. Hemi-central retinal vein occlusion is believed to be an anatomical variant of CRVO [8, 9]. Branch retinal vein occlusion (BRVO) involves one of the tributary veins of the retina.

Many systemic factors, such as diabetes, hypertension, and cardiovascular disease, have been associated with retinal vein occlusion [2, 4, 6, 10–20]. These factors are believed to affect vascular flow or cause vascular wall abnormalities, thereby contributing to the development of retinal vein occlusion. Most reports in the literature describe retinal vein occlusion in the face of specific systemic vascular diseases. However, studies implying increased prevalence of specific systemic vascular diseases in retinal vein occlusion rarely used adequate controls. It is uncertain whether any systemic vascular disease is actually more prevalent in retinal vein occlusion patients, thus, any relationship between the retinal vein occlusion and systemic diseases must be viewed with caution. In the absence of well-designed experimental studies or epidemiologic studies, the maxim, "Correlation does not imply causation," rings loud and clear. However, the presumed correlation of certain systemic diseases and retinal vein occlusion provides fertile ground for clinical investigation. Although the definitive picture remains to be established, existing pieces in the puzzle fit prevailing hypotheses used to explain the pathophysiology of retinal vein occlusion. These hypotheses remain unconfirmed, but the clinician can be guided to look for specific associated systemic conditions that may, in their own right, warrant treatment and that may influence the prognosis of the retinal vein occlusion.

Systemic Diseases and Central Retinal Vein Thrombosis

Systemic diseases may influence thrombus formation in the central retinal vein through (1) external compression, (2) primary thrombus formation through stasis, or (3) degenerative or inflammatory disorders of the vein itself.

Understanding the possible influence of various systemic diseases on the evolution of retinal vein occlusion requires knowledge of the unique anatomical arrangement of the retinal blood vessels in the eye as well as insight into the coagulation process.

When the vein enters the lamina cribrosa, the intraluminal pressure of the vein decreases, rendering it highly susceptible to collapse [21]. In addition, venomotor and vasomotor reflexes, which regulate the vascular tone, may lead to vasoconstriction and further decrease in the vessel lumen in the case of an outflow obstruction [22]. The central retinal artery shares a closed common compartment with the central retinal vein within the optic nerve. A space-occupying lesion within this space, such as arteriosclerotic or hypertensive changes in the artery, would compress the adjacent central retinal vein [21, 23]. These anatomical conditions predispose the central retinal vein to thrombus formation, which results in blood flow turbulence and slowing within the central retinal vein. The turbulence can shear off the intraluminal endothelial cells, setting in motion the clotting cascade. This process is exacerbated by blood flow slowing. CRVO has been reported in the face of central artery occlusion. This can be explained through stagnation of the retinal circulation brought about by partial or complete occlusion of the retinal artery, thereby precipitating secondary thrombus formation in the central retinal vein [24–26].

External compression from other conditions can create CRVO. Papilledema can lead to increased pressure within the optic nerve sheath and hence impinge on the central retinal vein [27]. Indeed, optic neuritis can, in rare instances, create sufficient intraaxonal swelling to impinge on the central retinal vein and produce a CRVO-like picture [28]. Ophthalmopathy, orbital tumors and abscesses, cavernous sinus thrombosis, and retrobulbar intranerve sheath injections are other rare conditions that can cause external compression on the optic nerve sheath and may precipitate a CRVO [29–35].

The anatomy of vasculature in the retina predisposes to BRVO. The artery shares a common adventitial sheath with the branch retinal vein [36]. Arteries crossing over veins anatomically contribute to the cause of BRVO. Conditions that increase the thickness of the crossing branch retinal artery wall would logically increase the likelihood of compression on the underlying branch retinal vein [37, 38].

These anatomical considerations also render the retinal venous system highly vulnerable to thrombus formation from hypercoagulable states, elevated viscosity, or systemic states of decreased thrombolysis. Intraocular retinal venous pressure must remain high to prevent the retinal veins from collapsing under high intraocular pressure. This elevated intraocular venous pressure is brought about through high resistance to flow in the central retinal vein, especially in the cribriform layer, where the central retinal artery and vein are closely approximated. However, this increased resistance limits the ability of the retinal venous circulation to adapt to increased blood viscosity. Retinal vein occlusion has been described in hyperviscosity syndromes such as hypergammaglobulinemia, paraproteinemia, hyperfibrinogenemia, and cryofibrinogenemia, as well as blood dyscrasias (leukemia, sickle cell disease, polycythemia vera, etc.) [16, 19, 30, 39–44]. Other conditions that affect the clotting cascade and create a potentially hypercoagulable state include protein S deficiency and external hormonal supplementation such as birth control pills [45]. Finally, increased platelet aggregability rounds out the effect on the blood coagulation system [46, 47].

Increased blood viscosity is believed to play an important contributory role in the development of retinal vein occlusion. Viscosity may be increased through blood cell volume or through changes that raise plasma viscosity. Of the two, blood cell volume is more important. Erythrocytes are believed to play a greater role than leukocytes or platelets by virtue of their larger numbers. Hemoglobin and packed red blood cell volume reflect the number of red blood cells. Piermarocchi and colleagues [48] showed a direct correlation between blood viscosity and hematocrit. In their study, blood viscosity was higher in patients with BRVO. Trope and co-workers [44] showed elevated blood viscosity and hematocrit in retinal vein occlusion patients when compared to controls. Ring and associates [19] also reported abnormal blood viscosity associated with elevated hematocrit in patients with retinal vein thrombosis. Chabanel and colleagues [49] suggested that increased erythrocyte aggregability and increased shear resistance of erythrocyte aggregability may contribute to the onset of retinal vascular occlusion by predisposing to circulatory stasis. A combination of low flow and vascular resistance within the central retinal vein might severely limit its ability to adjust to high blood viscosity. These findings were supported by Glacet-Bernard and co-workers [50].

Avins and Krummenacher [51] described venous stasis retinopathy in Gaisböck's syndrome, which is characterized by a decrease in plasma volume. A decrease in cell mass results in a relative increase in hematocrit. Despite the elevated hematocrit, viscosity in their patient was reported to be normal.

Plasma viscosity may also influence blood viscosity [19, 42–44, 48]. Raised erythrocyte sedimentation rate suggests raised plasma viscosity. Appiah and Trempe [8] found an association between elevated erythrocyte sedimentation rate of unknown cause and CRVO. Piermarocchi [48] showed that abnormal erythrocyte deformability can increase viscosity.

Whatever the cause, abnormal blood viscosity may contribute to thrombus formation at sites of low blood flow, such as at the level of an arterial venous crossing in BRVO or at the lamina cribrosa in CRVO. When blood flow is reduced, blood viscosity increases dramatically, primarily due to erythrocyte aggregation. Elevated fibrinogen or hematocrit favors this phenomenon. Furthermore, the hematocrit plays a greater role as the shear rate decreases. Thus, a decrease in blood flow at an anatomically predisposed site leads to a local and dramatic increase in blood viscosity, which further worsens the already compromised blood flow. This vicious spiral may lead to thrombus formation.

Systemic diseases such as malignancy, paraproteinemia, nephrotic syndrome, chronic lung disease, and Behçet's disease are all associated with elevated viscosity [52]. Primary macroglobulinemia, from plasma cell dyscrasia, typically results in a monoclonal IgM kappa protein that remains in the intravascular space [39]. Due to its pentametric shape, higher molecular weight, and tendency to aggregate, the IgM gammopathy leads to hyperviscosity. The macroglobulin also coats circulating erythrocytes leading to rouleaux formation. All these factors contribute to increased whole blood viscosity. Treatment involves plasmapheresis to reduce the hyperviscosity state by decreasing the serum IgM concentration and whole blood viscosity. Chemotherapy is used to control the underlying lymphoproliferative disorder.

Much interest has centered recently on deficiencies of circulating factors, which may lead to increased tendency for thrombus formation [53–55]. Antithrombin III, heparin co-factor II, platelet Factor III, protein C, and protein S act on the coagulation pathway. Fibrinolysis is mediated by prekallikrein and Factor XII, tissue plasminogen activator, and urokinase. Assays are available in most laboratories for the more common deficiencies: antithrombin III, protein C, and protein S. Recurrent thrombosis has been associated with homozygous protein C deficiency and protein S deficiency [56, 57].

Thrombosis has not yet been proved in heterozygous protein C deficiency. Chung and colleagues [58] suggested an association between protein C deficiency and BRVO but not CRVO.

Antiphospholipid antibodies are immunoglobulins seen in the antiphospholipid syndrome [59]. This may manifest as a primary entity, in the absence of any specific autoimmune disease, but more commonly is seen in association with systemic lupus erythematosus or lupuslike disease. These antibodies interfere with endothelial cells and prevent interaction of natural anticoagulants and platelets, thereby encouraging thrombosis. An association with retinal vein occlusion has been suggested [60–62].

Primary diseases of the vessels may explain the pathogenesis of retinal vein occlusion, perhaps through an interaction on the clotting system. Infectious vasculitis (tuberculosis, syphilis, the acquired immunodeficiency syndrome [AIDS]) and systemic vascular disorders such as connective tissue diseases have been associated with retinal vein occlusion [63]. Silverman and co-workers [64] reported a patient with CRVO and systemic lupus erythematosus who had a prolonged partial thromboplastin time, suggesting the presence of lupus anticoagulant. Tolosa-Vilella and colleagues [65] reported 2 cases of BRVO and primary antiphospholipid syndrome.

Ruby and Jampol [66] described several cases of Crohn's disease with retinal vein occlusion. They suggest that increased plasma fibrin peptide A levels and increased production of monocyte tissue factor may contribute to the activation of blood coagulation in Crohn's patients [67]. Furthermore, plasma in patients with inflammatory bowel disease shows decreased tissue type plasminogen activator activity, increased plasminogen activator and fibrinogen, and prolonged thrombin and prothrombin times.

Retinal vein occlusion may also occur as the result of localized inflammation of the involved vein. An example of this is sarcoid [68–70]. Periphlebitis resulting in retinal vein occlusion may also occasionally be seen in serpiginous choroiditis [71, 72]. Friberg [72] speculates that the perivascular response seen in these patients may result from antigen-antibody interactions in the vessel wall rather than from extension of choroidal inflammation into the retinal layers. Charteris and colleagues [73] reported a case of CRVO and acute posterior multifocal placoid pigment epitheliopathy. They suggest an underlying systemic vasculitis. Leung and associates [74] reported a clinicopathological case of polyarteritis presenting with thrombocytosis and CRVO. They were unable to determine whether the retinal vein occlusion resulted from vasculitis or a hypercoagulable state.

Rock and associates [45] reported retinal periphlebitis after hormonal treatment in 2 cases. One case involved a healthy 31-year-old male treated with clomiphene, an antiestrogenic drug. The second case involved a 32-year-old healthy woman on oral contraceptives for 5 years prior to the onset of venous occlusive disease.

Evaluation of Systemic Disease Risk in the Presence of CRVO

My colleagues and I recently reviewed the risk for systemic vascular diseases in patients with CRVO [13]. In this cross-sectional study, 197 patients in whom CRVO was diagnosed at the Wilmer Ophthalmological Institute between 1980 and 1985 were compared with National Health Interview Survey (NHIS) patients and Wilmer cataract patients. The prevalence of hypertension was significantly elevated in the CRVO cases when compared with both comparison groups ($p < .03$, .005). Prevalence of diabetes mellitus was increased in CRVO cases in comparison with the NHIS group ($p < .005$). The prevalence of cerebrovascular or cardiovascular disease was the same for all three groups. The discrepancy for diabetes between the expected NHIS rates and the Wilmer controls can be explained by two factors: (1) The Wilmer control group represents a hospital population attending tertiary care centers and, thus, may have an increased prevalence of diabetes mellitus compared with the healthy population, and (2) since cataracts are associated with diabetes mellitus, the Wilmer controls may have an increased prevalence of diabetes mellitus.

Based on our cross-sectional study, as well as a review of the literature, several medical recommendations can be offered. Patients with CRVO should be evaluated for hypertension and diabetes. As the prevalence of cerebrovascular and cardiovascular disease is not significantly higher in patients with CRVO, routine diagnostic procedures that test cardiac function, coronary artery patency, and cerebrovascular blood flow do not seem warranted unless specifically indicated otherwise. More aggressive systemic workup, particularly hematological, appears warranted when bilateral retinal vascular disease presents. However, most retinal vein occlusions appear to be idiopathic.

References

1. Brown GC, Brown RH, Brown MM. Peripheral proliferative retinopathies. Int Ophthalmol 1987;11:41–50
2. Quinlan PM, Elman MJ, Bhatt AK, et al. The natural course of central retinal vein occlusion. Am J Ophthalmol 1990;110(2):118–123
3. Rubinstein K, Jones EB. Retinal vein occlusion: long-term prospects—10 years' follow-up of 143 patients. Br J Ophthalmol 1976;60:148–150
4. Sedney SC. Photocoagulation in retinal vein occlusion. Doc Ophthalmol 1976;40: 1–241
5. Walters RF, Spalton DJ. Central retinal vein occlusion in people aged 40 years or less: a review of 17 patients. Br J Ophthalmol 1990;74:30–35
6. Zegarra H, Gutman FA, Conforto J. The natural course of central retinal vein occlusion. Ophthalmology 1979;86:1931–1939

7. Green WR, Chan CC, Hutchins GM, Terry JM. Central retinal vein occlusion: a prospective histopathologic study of 29 eyes in 28 cases. Retina 1981;1:27–55
8. Appiah AP, Trempe CL. Differences in contributory factors among hemicentral, central, and branch retinal vein occlusions. Ophthalmology 1989;96:364–366
9. Appiah AP, Trempe CL. Risk factors associated with branch vs. central retinal vein occlusion. Ann Ophthalmol 1989;21:153–157
10. Appiah PA, Greenidge KC. Factors associated with retinal-vein occlusion in Hispanics. Ann Ophthalmol 1987;19:307–312
11. Cassidy VJ. Central retinal vein thrombosis. Am J Ophthalmol 1953;36:331–335
12. Dodson PM, Galton DJ, Hamilton AM, Black RK. Retinal vein occlusion and the prevalence of lipoprotein abnormalities. Br J Ophthalmol 1982;66:161–164
13. Elman MJ, Bhatt AK, Quinlan PM, Enger C. The risk of systemic vascular diseases and mortality in patients with central retinal vein occlusion. Ophthalmology 1990; 97:11
14. Kohner EM, Laatikainen L, Oughton J. The management of central retinal vein occlusion. Ophthalmology 1983;90:484–487
15. Kohner EM, Cappin JM. Do medical conditions have an influence on central retinal vein occlusion? Proc R Soc Med 1974;67:1052–1054
16. McGrath MA, Wechsler F, Hunyor ABL, Penny R. Systemic factors contributory to retinal vein occlusion. Arch Intern Med 1978;138:216–220
17. Paton A, Rubinstein K, Smith VH. Arterial insufficiency in retinal venous occlusion (a short symposium). Trans Ophthalmol Soc UK 1964;84:559–595
18. Priluck IA, Robertson DM, Hollenhorst RW. Long-term follow-up of occlusion of the central retinal vein in young adults. Am J Ophthalmol 1980;90:190–202
19. Ring CP, Pearson TC, Saunders MD, Wetherley-Mein G. Viscosity and retinal vein thrombosis. Br J Ophthalmol 1976;60:397–410
20. Saraux H, Pelosse B. Long-term follow-up and etiologic factors in edematous forms of central retinal vein obstruction. J Fr Ophtalmol 1989;12:339–341
21. Verhoeff FH. Obstruction of central retinal vein. Arch Ophthalmol 1907;36:1–36
22. Behrman S. Retinal vein obstruction. Br J Ophthalmol 1962;46:336–342
23. Klien BA, Olwin JH. A survey of the pathogenesis of retinal venous occlusion. Arch Ophthalmol 1956;56:207–247
24. Duker JS, Cohen MS, Brown GC, et al. Combined branch retinal artery and central retinal vein obstruction. Retina 1990;10:105–112
25. Noble MJ, Alvarez EV. Combined occlusion of the central retinal artery and central retinal vein following blunt ocular trauma: a case report. Br J Ophthalmol 1987; 71:834–836
26. Richards RD. Simultaneous occlusion of the central retinal artery and vein. Trans Am Ophthalmol Soc 1979;77:191–199
27. Kwann HC, Dobbie JG. Thromboembolic disorders of the eye. In: Kwann HC, Bowie EJW, eds. Thrombosis. Philadelphia: Saunders, 1982:107–113
28. Duker JS, Sergott RC, Savino PJ, Bosley TM. Optic neuritis with secondary retinal venous stasis. Ophthalmology 1989;96:475–480
29. Brunette I, Boghen D. Central retinal vein occlusion complicating spontaneous carotid-cavernous fistula. Case report. Arch Ophthalmol 1987;105:464–465
30. Gutman FA. Evaluation of a patient with central retinal vein occlusion. Ophthalmology 1983;90:481–483
31. Hashimoto M, Yokota A, Matsuoka S, et al. Central retinal vein occlusion after treatment of cavernous dural arteriovenous malformation. AJNR 1989;10(5 suppl): S30-1
32. Komiyama M, Yamanakia K, Nagata Y, Ishikawa H. Dural carotid-cavernous sinus fistula and central retinal vein occlusion: a case report and a review of the literature. Surg Neurol 1990;34:255–259

33. Morgan CM, Schatz H, Vine AK, et al. Ocular complications associated with retrobulbar injections. Ophthalmology 1988;95:660–665
34. Pollack S, Miller NR. Central retinal vein occlusion complicating spontaneous carotid-cavernous fistula. Arch Ophthalmol 1986;104:331
35. Suzuki Y, Kase M, Yokoi M, et al. Development of central retinal vein occlusion in dural carotid-cavernous fistula. Ophthalmologica 1989;199:28–33
36. Michaelson IC. The pathogenesis of retinal branch vein occlusion. Doc Ophthalmol Proc Ser 1974;5:125–130
37. Duker JS, Brown GC. Anterior location of the crossing artery in branch retinal vein obstruction. Arch Ophthalmol 1989;107:998–1000
38. Weinberg D, Dogwell DG, Fern SA. Anatomy of arteriovenous crossings in branch retinal vein occlusion. Am J Ophthalmol 1990;109:298–302
39. Avashia JH, Fath DF. Bilateral central retinal vein occlusion in Waldenstrom's macroglobulinemia. J Am Optom Assoc 1989;60:657–658
40. Kienast J, Vermylen J, Verstraete M. Venous thromboses in particular organs. J Am Coll Cardiol 1986;8(6 suppl B):137B–145B
41. McGrath MA, Penny R, Wechsler F, Hunyor ABL. The pathogenesis of retinal vein thrombosis (abstr). Aust NZ J Med 1973;3:329
42. Peduzzi M, Codeluppi L, Poggi M, et al. Abnormal blood viscosity and erythrocyte deformability in retinal vein occlusion. Am J Ophthalmol 1983;96:399–400
43. Peduzzi M, Debbia A, Guerrieri F, et al. Abnormal blood rheology in retinal vein occlusion. A preliminary report. Graefes Arch Clin Exp Ophthalmol 1986;224: 83–85
44. Trope GE, Lowe GDO, McArdle BM, et al. Abnormal blood viscosity and haemostasis in long standing retinal vein occlusion. Br J Ophthalmol 1983;67:137–142
45. Rock T, Dinar Y, Romem M. Retinal periphlebitis after hormonal treatment. Ann Ophthalmol 1989;21:75–76
46. De Rosa V, Peduzzi M, Coccheri S. Haemostasis in retinal vein occlusion: fibrinolytic response and recanalization (abstr). Thromb Haemost 1979;42:208
47. Priluck IA. Impending central retinal vein occlusion associated with increased platelet aggregability. Ann Ophthalmol 1979;11:79–84
48. Piermarocchi S, Segato T, Bertoja H, et al. Branch retinal vein occlusion: the pathogenetic role of blood viscosity. Ann Ophthalmol 1990;22:303–311
49. Chabanel A, Glacet-Bernard A, Lelong F, et al. Increased red blood cell aggregation in retinal vein occlusion. Br J Haematol 1990;75:127–131
50. Glacet-Bernard A, Coscas G, Lelong F, et al. Erythrocyte aggregation and retinal vein occlusion. Preliminary data for a randomized study on the efficacy of anti-erythrocyte aggregation (troxerutin) in retinal vein occlusion. Bull Soc Ophtalmol Fr 1989;89:1393–1396
51. Avins LR, Krummenacher TK. Venous stasis retinopathy and Gaisbock's syndrome. Am J Ophthalmol 1988;105:420–421
52. Graham EM. The investigation of patients with retinal vascular occlusion. Eye 1990;4(pt 3):464–468
53. Favilla I, Stubbs K, Kowal L. Abnormal fibrinolysis in retinal vein occlusion. Aust J Ophthalmol 1981;9:213–218
54. Gum KB, Carter KD, Vine AK. Massive bilateral retinal vascular occlusion secondary to thrombotic thrombocytopenic purpura. Retina 1988;8:185–187
55. Patrassi GM, Mares M, Piermarocchi S, et al. Fibrinolytic behavior in long-standing branch retinal vein occlusion. Ophthalmic Res 1987;19:221–225
56. Comp PC, Esmon CT. Recurrent venous thrombo-embolism in patients with partial deficiency of protein S. N Engl J Med 1984;311:1525–1528
57. Seligsohn U, Berger A, Abend M, et al. Homozygous protein C deficiency manifested by massive venous thrombosis in the newborn. N Engl J Med 1984;310: 559–562

58. Chung MM, Trese MT, Hong YJ. Protein C levels in retinal vein occlusions. Invest Ophthalmol Vis Sci 1989;30(suppl):477
59. Asherson RA, Merry P, Acheson JF, et al. Antiphospholipid antibodies: a risk factor for occlusive ocular vascular disease in systemic lupus erythematosus and the "primary" antiphospholipid syndrome. Ann Rheum Dis 1989;48:358–361
60. Fitzpatrick EP, Chesen N, Rahn EK. The lupus anticoagulant and retinal vasoocclusive disease. Ann Ophthalmol 1990;22:148–152
61. Heckerling PS, Froelich CJ, Schade SG. Retinal vein thrombosis in a patient with pernicious anemia and anticardiolipin antibodies. J Rheumatol 1989;16:1144–1146
62. Pulido JS, Ward LM, Fishman GA, et al. Antiphospholipid antibodies associated with retinal vascular disease. Retina 1987;7:215–218
63. Teich SA, Sonnabend J. Central retinal vein occlusion in a patient with AIDS. Case report. Arch Ophthalmol 1988;106:1508–1509
64. Silverman H, Lubeck MJ, Briney WG. Central retinal vein occlusion complicating systemic lupus erythematosus. Arthritis Rheum 1978;21:839–843
65. Tolosa-Vilella C, Ordi-Ros J, Jordana-Comajuneosa R, et al. Occlusive ocular vascular disease and anti-phospholipid antibodies. Ann Rheum Dis 1990;49:203
66. Ruby AJ, Jampol LM. Crohn's disease and retinal vascular disease. Am J Ophthalmol 1990;110(4):349–353
67. Edwards RL, Levine JL, Green R, et al. Activation of blood coagulation in Crohn's disease. Gastroenterology 1987;92:329
68. Gass JDM, Olson CL. Sarcoidosis with optic nerve and retinal involvement. Arch Ophthalmol 1976;94:945
69. Kimmel AS, McCarthy MJ, Blodi CF, Folk JC. Branch retinal vein occlusion in sarcoidosis. Am J Ophthalmol 1989;107:561–562
70. Sanders MD, Shilling JS. Retinal, choroidal, and optic disc involvement in sarcoidosis. Trans Ophthalmol Soc (UK) 1976;96:140–144
71. Blumenkranz MS, Gass JDM, Clarkson JG. A typical serpiginous choroiditis. Arch Ophthalmol 1982;100:1773
72. Friberg TR. Serpiginous choroiditis with branch vein occlusion and bilateral periphlebitis. Case report. Arch Ophthalmol 1988;106:585–586
73. Charteris DG, Khanna V, Dhillon B. Acute posterior multifocal placoid pigment epitheliopathy complicated by central retinal vein occlusion. Br J Ophthalmol 1989;73:765–768
74. Leung AC, McLay A, Boulton-Jones JM. Polyarteritis presenting with thrombocytosis and central retinal vein thrombosis. Scott Med J 1987;32:24–26

Systemic Associations of Retinal Vasculitis

Miles R. Stanford, F.R.C.S.
Elizabeth M. Graham, M.R.C.P.

Retinal vasculitis may be broadly defined as inflammation within the eye that involves the retinal vessels. It is usually a disorder that affects young people and gives rise to significant visual morbidity [1]. It may be associated with infections, ischemia, or malignancy but, in a majority of cases, the cause of the disorder is unknown and confined to the eye or is present as part of a multisystem inflammatory disorder [2]. There is increasing evidence from both human and animal work that these idiopathic forms represent an organ-specific autoimmune disorder against ocular antigens [3]. From the clinical point of view, very few of these diseases show pathognomonic retinal features so that the identification of the underlying disease must come from systemic evaluation. However, it is worth identifying the retinal vessels that are predominantly involved, whether arteries, veins, or capillaries, as this helps to define the differential diagnosis (Table) [4]. In this review, we do not propose to discuss those diseases for which there is an obvious cause (infections or malignancy) but will concentrate on the associated systemic features of idiopathic disease and try to relate these to the ocular findings.

Polyarteritis Nodosa

Polyarteritis nodosa (PAN) may affect every tissue of the eye. Retinal vascular involvement is primarily arterial and gives rise to cotton-wool spots, retinal edema, and hypertensive changes. Vitritis is rare [5].

PAN is an arteritis that causes inflammation of all three coats of medium-sized muscular arteries. Deposition of immunoglobulin and complement fixation may be demonstrated in these vessel walls, and the pathological consequences are aneurysm formation, thrombosis, and infarction. The process may affect any part of the body, but kidney, heart, brain, and gastrointestinal tract are the common sites.

Clinically, early features are nonspecific and consist of fever, malaise, weight loss, arthralgia, and skin rashes. Renal involvement is found in 75% of patients and leads to hypertension, proteinuria, hematuria, and renal failure.

Correlation of Retinal Features of Systemic Inflammatory Disease with Size of Vessel Involved

Vessel Involved	Disease	Retinal Features
Muscular arteries	Polyarteritis nodosa	Cotton-wool spots, retinal edema, hypertensive changes
Medium to small arteries	Wegener's granulomatosis	Cotton-wool spots, arteriolar occlusion
Small arteries	Systemic lupus erythematosus	Cotton-wool spots, hemorrhage, retinal edema, new vessels
Capillaries	Whipple's disease	Hemorrhage, exudate, capillary occlusion
Veins	Behçet's disease	Infiltrates, branch vein occlusions, macular edema, neovascularization
	Sarcoidosis	Periphlebitis, venous sheathing, choroidal granuloma, neovascularization
	Multiple sclerosis	Venous sheathing, macular edema, neovascularization
Arteries and veins	Crohn's disease	Vascular occlusions
	Polychondritis	Exudate and hemorrhage
Miscellaneous	Ankylosing spondylitis, HLA-B27-positive	Macular edema, vitritis, diffuse microvascular leakage

Angiographic evidence of multiple aneurysms in the kidney is almost pathognomonic. Cardiac involvement occurs in 80% and may give rise to myocardial infarction, coronary arteritis, and acute pericarditis. Sixty percent of patients show mononeuritis multiplex and often have a mixed sensory and motor neuropathy. Cerebral manifestations include psychosis, hemiparesis, and brainstem lesions. Abdominal pain or an acute abdomen is a well-known presentation of PAN. Any abdominal organ may be affected by secondary ischemia, with the development of bloody diarrhea being an ominous sign. Pulmonary involvement in classical PAN is rare. Up to 40% of patients are hepatitis B–positive.

The prognosis for PAN is fairly good, with 80% of patients surviving for 5 years. Treatment is with high-dose steroids and immunosuppressive agents. There is good evidence that if patients can be treated successfully through their illness, relapse is very uncommon.

■ Wegener's Granulomatosis

The eye is affected in up to 50% of patients with Wegener's granulomatosis. This usually results in proptosis secondary to orbital granulomas, or scleritis. However, retinal vasculitis has been reported and is represented by varying degrees of arteriolar occlusion leading to cotton-wool spots and retinal edema [6]. The rare nonsarcoidal variant of Wegener's granulomatosis has the same retinal features as sarcoidosis (see page 26).

The disease is a rare form of necrotizing vasculitis that usually affects the small vessels of the lung and upper respiratory tract with glomerulonephritis. Men are more affected than women, and patients are usually older than 40 years. The most common presentation is with chronic sinusitis and rhinorrhea. Lung involvement is often asymptomatic but may present as acute bronchitis or, more rarely, hemoptysis. Nodules, infiltrates, and cavitation may be seen on roentgenography. Glomerulonephritis occurs in 85% of patients and is progressive, leading to renal failure and death if untreated. Serological examination often reveals a raised anti–neutrophil cytoplasm antibody (ANCA) titer and a polyclonal increase in immunoglobulins. Cyclophosphamide is the drug of choice, although other immunosuppressives may be efficacious.

■ Systemic Lupus Erythematosus

Systemic lupus erythematosus (SLE) is a multisystem disorder that may affect all coats of the eye. Retinal vascular involvement is primarily arterial, giving rise to cotton-wool spots, retinal edema, and neovascularization [7]. Vitritis is uncommon. The recognition of lupus retinopathy is important as it signifies major activity of the underlying disease.

SLE affects women more than men and is more common in the young and in Negroes. The underlying pathological process is a systemic vasculitis with fibrinoid necrosis occurring in small arteries that is probably secondary to immune complex deposition in the vessel wall. These changes are found in all arterioles, including those of the retina and choroid [8].

SLE may affect all parts of the body. The most common symptom is an arthralgia, but erosive arthritis is unusual. Cutaneous manifestations include the characteristic butterfly rash across the face or, more commonly, discoid lupus with hyperkeratosis and fibrinoid necrosis in the dermis. Often, these rashes are photosensitive. Central nervous system (CNS) involvement is a major problem in SLE, occurring in 60% of patients. Features include seizures, hemiplegia, ataxia, aseptic meningitis, and cranial nerve lesions. Psychiatric problems range from mild depression to progressive dementia.

Renal involvement in SLE occurs in at least 50% of patients and leads to hypertension and renal failure. In the lung pleurisy, pleural effusion and elevation of the diaphragm may be seen. Pericarditis or a mild myocarditis are common cardiac lesions, with the classical lesion of mitral valve vegetations (Libman-Sacks disease) being extremely rare and usually only found at autopsy.

Hematological and immunological abnormalities are common. Varying degrees of anemia, leukopenia, or thrombocytopenia are seen, and high titers of antibody to double-stranded DNA are characteristic. There may also be a polyclonal hypergammaglobulinemia, raised circulating immune complexes, reduced serum complement, and a positive rheumatoid factor.

The disease responds to systemic corticosteroids, but minor forms may be controlled with nonsteroidal antiinflammatory agents. Chloroquine salts are useful for maintaining remission but require ophthalmological supervision. Occasionally, systemic immunosuppressives such as azathioprine or cyclophosphamide are required to control renal disease or as steroid-sparing agents.

■ Whipple's Disease

The eye is rarely involved in Whipple's disease. Retinal vascular damage is seen at the capillary level, leading to hemorrhage, exudates, and capillary occlusion. Choroidal folds have also been reported [9].

Systemic disease is dominated by intestinal involvement that leads to malabsorption. The patient may present with malaise, weight loss, diarrhea, and arthritis—the latter being migratory, nonerosive, and usually affecting peripheral joints. Extraintestinal disease may include pleurisy with pulmonary infiltrates, pericarditis, ascites, cardiac conduction defects, and myopathy—but all these are usually due to secondary nutritional deficiencies consequent to malabsorption. CNS involvement with dementia, eye movement disorders including supranuclear ophthalmoplegia, ataxia, and myoclonus may also be seen.

The disease is characterized pathologically by macrophages containing gram-negative bacteria that stain intensely with periodic acid–Schiff reagent. Treatment is empirical, but the disease usually responds to tetracycline, and therefore the diagnosis should always be considered in undiagnosed cases of retinal vasculitis.

■ Sarcoidosis

Sarcoidosis, a multisystem disorder of unknown etiology, most commonly affects young adults and usually presents with bilateral hilar lymphadenopathy (BHL) and ocular and skin lesions. While there are no pathognomonic retinal features of sarcoidosis, periphlebitis is characteristic, and venous sheathing, macular edema, choroidal granulomas, and neovascularization may also be seen [10]. Optic disc swelling may arise secondary to uveitis, raised intracranial pressure, or optic nerve infiltration.

Sarcoid granulomas may be present in every organ system of the body. These are characteristically noncaseating and associated with giant cells. BHL is usually found in acute disease and is often asymptomatic (Fig 1). Pulmonary infiltration rarely causes symptoms, but progressive pulmonary fibrosis leads to a restrictive ventilatory defect. Surprisingly, this latter form of disease is rarely associated with retinal vasculitis, although cicatricial conjunctival changes have been reported.

The other main organ affected in sarcoidosis is the skin. Erythema nodosum is an early feature of acute disease and generally reflects a favorable prognosis (Fig 2). Sarcoid infiltration, especially in old scars, may occur anywhere in the skin with the red induration of the nose (lupus pernio) being characteristic. Arthropathy is usually transient and mild, but a persistent polyarthritis may be seen in widespread disease.

Other organs may be infiltrated with sarcoid granulomas. Biopsy-proved infiltration of the liver occurs in 70% of patients with active disease. Though

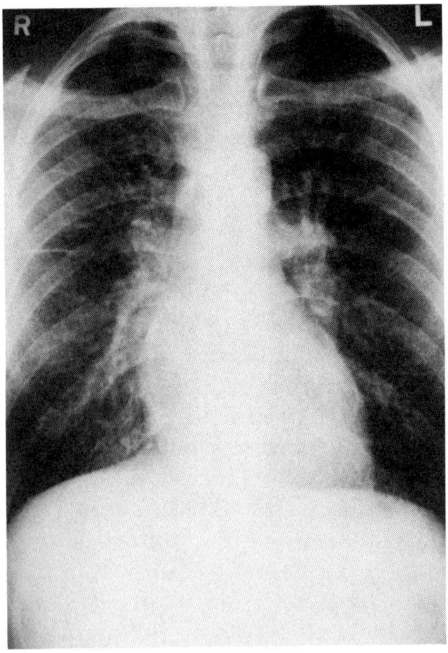

Figure 1 *Posteroanterior chest roentgenogram from a 30-year-old man with sarcoidosis. Note bilateral hilar lymphadenopathy and nodular infiltrates.*

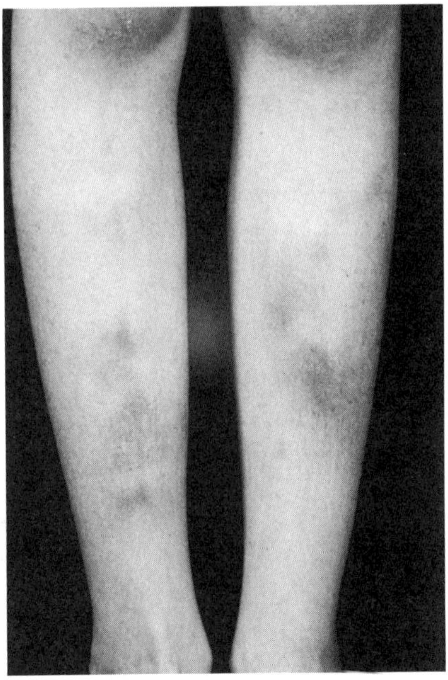

Figure 2 *Erythema nodosum presents as red, slightly tender, raised plaques over the shins.*

this rarely gives rise to signs, chronic fibrosis may lead to jaundice and portal hypertension. Mild to moderate splenomegaly may occur, which is usually secondary to hepatic disease. The kidney may become infiltrated in chronic active disease, but renal failure usually results from hypercalcemia and hypercalciuria. Lymphadenopathy is common. Muscular infiltration may lead to a proximal myopathy. Rarely, myocardial granulomas give rise to conduction defects and arrhythmias leading to sudden death. CNS disease leads to cranial nerve palsies, most commonly of the face, with other manifestations depending on the site of the granuloma (e.g., optic nerve, brainstem). Involvement of the parotid and lacrimal glands leads initially to swelling and then to a reduction in function.

The diagnosis of sarcoidosis depends on clinical suspicion. Blood tests may show a lymphopenia, a diffuse rise in gamma globulins, a raised erythrocyte sedimentation rate and serum angiotensin-converting enzyme level, and variable changes in biochemical values such as hypercalcemia and abnormal liver and renal function tests. Uptake of radioactive gallium by granulomas may be demonstrated. The Mantoux reaction is often negative. Granulomas may be demonstrated by conjunctival biopsy in 50%, transbronchial biopsy in 70%, and by the Kveim test in 80%.

The majority of the manifestations of sarcoid are transient and require no specific treatment. Life-threatening infiltration requires corticosteroid therapy, often long-term. Retinal vasculitis may be controlled with systemic steroids, azathioprine, or cyclophosphamide.

■ Behçet's Disease

Behçet's disease, a chronic inflammatory disorder, classically presents with recurrent orogenital ulceration and ocular, neurological, skin, or arthritic changes. The most common ocular manifestation is recurrent anterior uveitis with hypopyon, but retinal vasculitis is the major cause of visual morbidity. Retinal infiltrates are characteristic and are not seen in any other idiopathic retinal vasculitis. Inflammatory retinal vein occlusions, macular edema, neovascularization, optic disc swelling, and eventual optic atrophy occur [11].

Recurrent orogenital ulceration is the hallmark of Behçet's disease, with mouth ulcers being more common (Fig 3). These resemble aphthous ulcers but may be very widespread and painful. They usually heal spontaneously

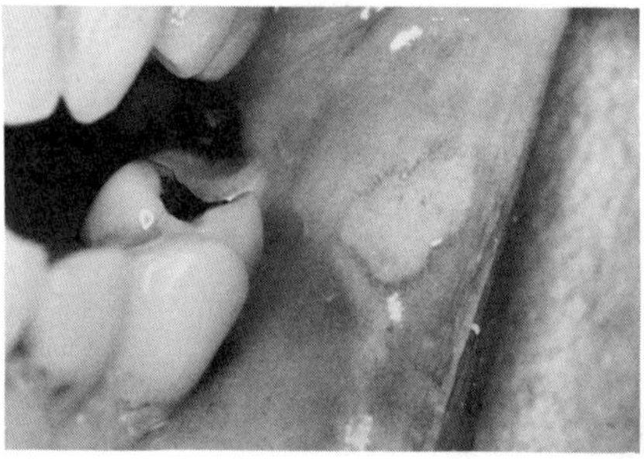

Figure 3 *Buccal mucosa of a 24-year-old woman with Behçet's disease showing ulceration. These ulcers typically heal without scarring.*

without scarring. Conversely, genital ulcers tend to be deep and leave a scar when they heal.

Skin lesions are common. These may resemble erythema nodosum or be acneiform. Again, they heal spontaneously without ulceration. Cutaneous hypersensitivity (dermatographia), pustular lesions at the site of trauma (the pathergy reaction), and superficial thrombophlebitis are also seen.

Less common manifestations of disease are arthropathy, vascular occlusions, and CNS involvement. Half the patients will have a nondestructive arthritis, usually affecting the knee, and this may be exacerbated when the disease becomes active. Vascular involvement presents as recurrent thrombophlebitis of the leg, vena caval obstruction, benign intracranial hypertension secondary to cerebral venous thrombosis, and coronary artery occlusion. Neurological Behçet's disease usually carries a poor prognosis and seems not to be associated with ocular disease. The brainstem, basal ganglion, and thalamus are involved, and frank psychiatric symptoms are common.

The etiology of Behçet's disease has been variously ascribed to allergic, viral, or genetic factors [12]. Pathologically, lesions show a central perivasculitis with tissue destruction around the vessel wall. Similar changes have been seen in the eye [13].

Behçet's disease responds to a variety of drugs, with corticosteroids being the mainstay of treatment. Additional drugs that are effective in controlling ocular disease are cyclosporine A, colchicine, and azathioprine; although, despite high doses of all these, some patients continue to lose sight.

■ Multiple Sclerosis

Retinal vasculitis is becoming an increasingly recognized complication of multiple sclerosis. Sporadic reports of peripheral venous sheathing have appeared in the literature [14], but not until recently has the true prevalence of this complication become apparent [15, 16]. The retinal vasculitis consists of peripheral venous sheathing, vitritis, macular edema and, rarely, neovascularization with vitreous hemorrhage [10]. The recognition of ocular disease is important as it may precede development of neurological signs and appears to signify a worse prognosis. Furthermore, the occurrence of vasculitis in a tissue that lacks myelin has pathogenetic significance, supporting the concept of a primarily vasculitic rather than myelinodestructive process causing disease in these patients.

The systemic presentation of multiple sclerosis may be extremely diverse, but the usual symptoms are related to lesions occurring in the optic nerve, brainstem, or spinal cord. However, there is good evidence from nuclear magnetic resonance studies that clinically silent lesions, especially in the periventricular white matter, may be extensive on presentation [17].

The clinical course of multiple sclerosis is varied, ranging from the patient with repeated relapse and remission to the one with a steadily progressive disability. In the remitting form, there is usually almost complete recovery after each attack but multiple attacks slowly lead to severe disability. Bad prognostic signs include late age at onset, progressive disease from the outset, or severe brainstem or spinal cord lesions at any age.

There is no specific treatment for multiple sclerosis. Steroids in high dosage limit the severity of individual attacks by reducing inflammation and its associated edema. Treatment of ocular disease is dependent on whether complications such as macular edema or neovascularization supervene.

■ Ankylosing Spondylitis

The most common ocular feature of ankylosing spondylitis is acute anterior uveitis. A few patients will develop a severe retinal vasculitis with chronic vitritis and macular edema, these usually having the HLA-B27 haplotype.

Ankylosing spondylitis usually occurs in young men, although women may also be affected. The classical presentation is low back pain on waking that is gradually relieved by exercise. As the disease progresses, pain may be experienced at higher levels in the spine. The disease may burn out at any stage, and few patients progress to total spinal ankylosis (Fig 4). An asymmetrical polyarthritis affecting the hip, knee, wrist, and shoulder but sparing the small joints of the hand and feet may occur. Neurological complications are usually related to spinal involvement, either from traumatic fractures or a cauda equina syndrome. Rare complications of this disorder include aortic incompetence from an aortitis, aneurysm formation, pulmonary fibrosis, and secondary amyloidosis leading to uremia.

The etiology of ankylosing spondylitis is unknown. A genetic susceptibility seems apparent in that 90% of patients possess the HLA-B27 haplotype, and there seems to be an association with gastrointestinal or genitourinary infections [18]. Retinal vasculitis often requires high doses of systemic steroids in the acute phase, and azathioprine is beneficial in reducing relapses. The skeletal problems may be managed with nonsteroidal antiinflammatory agents and the appropriate physiotherapy.

■ Crohn's Disease

Retinal vasculitis associated with Crohn's disease is rare, but some cases with occlusive arteritis and phlebitis have been reported [19]. Crohn's disease is a chronic inflammatory disease of the gastrointestinal tract that is frequently discontinuous and tends to cause fistulas. Most patients present with fever, diarrhea, abdominal pain, and weight loss depending on which part of the bowel is involved. Secondary changes such as anemia, osteomalacia, or bleeding tendencies are usually due to nutritional deficiencies from malabsorption. Interestingly, the extraintestinal manifestations of this disease show considerable overlap with other diseases associated with retinal vasculitis. Thus, recurrent aphthous ulceration, erythema nodosum, and arthritis are common (Fig 5) and relate to underlying disease activity. Sacroiliitis, ankylosing spondylitis, and liver changes also occur but tend to be independent of the disease.

Systemic corticosteroids are required for active disease, and surgical resection of involved bowel is required at least once in 80% of patients. Ocular disease responds to corticosteroids, and cyclophosphamide has also been used with good effect.

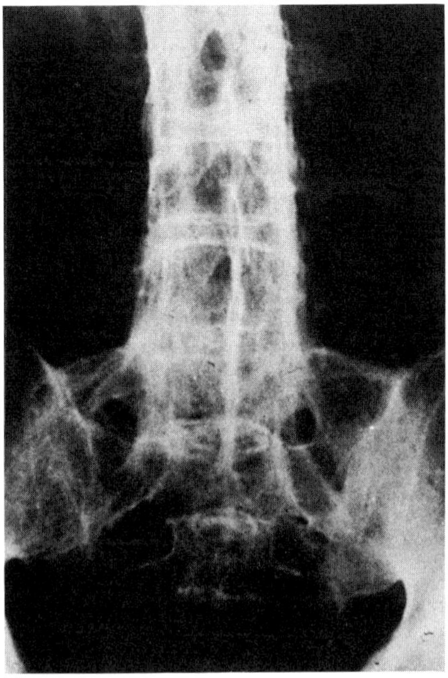

Figure 4 *Roentgenogram of lumbar spine of a 40-year-old man with ankylosing spondylitis. Note sclerosis of the sacroiliac joints and ankylosis of the lumbar vertebrae.*

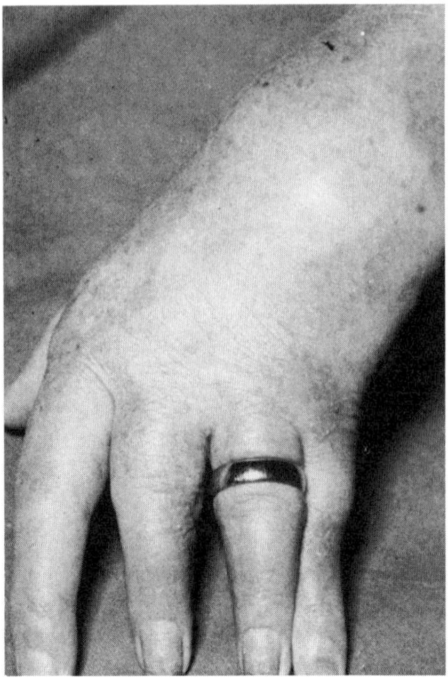

Figure 5 *Hand of a patient with a seronegative arthropathy (associated with Crohn's disease). Proximal interphalangeal joints are mainly involved.*

Relapsing Polychondritis

Ocular signs may be found in up to 60% of patients with relapsing polychondritis at some point in their illness. A retinal vasculitis has been described in 9% of patients with this rare disorder, consisting of exudates, hemorrhage, vascular occlusion, and serous detachments [20].

The disease is a systemic inflammatory disorder that affects the mucopolysaccharide component of the ground substance of cartilage. Untreated, it carries a high mortality. Involvement of ear and nasal cartilage leads to recurrent swelling and redness and eventual destruction. More serious is tracheal involvement leading to stridor, and aortic valve disease with aneurysm formation. Fever, malaise, vasculitis, and arthropathy may also occur at various stages.

Comments

It is important to recognize the associated clinical features that may occur in patients with retinal vasculitis and a systemic inflammatory disease. In our experience, only those patients with symptoms or signs of such a disease are likely to benefit from systemic investigation; although, in the case of multiple sclerosis, this may not always be true. Furthermore, the age of the patient (ocular ischemia and lymphoma are important causes of uveitis in patients older than 60) and the type of vessel involved should be carefully considered. The systemic associations of this disorder are important in unraveling the pathogenesis of ocular disease, because the underlying pathological process affecting the rest of the body appears, for the most part, to be occurring in the vessels of the eye as well.

This work was supported by the Iris Fund for the Prevention of Blindness.

References

1. Nussenblatt RB, Palestine AG. Uveitis: fundamentals and clinical practice. Chicago: Year Book, 1989
2. Sanders MD. Retinal arteritis, retinal vasculitis and autoimmune retinal vasculitis. Eye 1987;1:441–465
3. Gery I, Mochizuki M, Nussenblatt RB. Retinal specific antigens and immunopathogenic processes they provoke. In: Osborne N, Chader J, eds. Progress in retinal research. Oxford: Pergamon Press, 1986:75–109
4. James DG, Graham E, Hamblin A. Immunology of multisystem ocular disease. Surv Ophthalmol 1985;30:155–167
5. Morgan CM, Foster CS, Gragondas ES. Retinal vasculitis in polyarteritis nodosa. Retina 1986;6:205–209
6. Spalton DJ, Graham EM, Page NER, Sanders MD. Ocular changes in limited forms of Wegener's granulomatosis. Br J Ophthalmol 1981;65:553–563

7. Jabs DA, Fine SL, Hochberg MC, et al. Severe retinal vaso-occlusive disease in systemic lupus erythematosus. Arch Ophthalmol 1986;104:558–563
8. Graham EM, Spalton DJ, Barnard RO, et al. Cerebral and retinal changes in systemic lupus erythematosus. Ophthalmology 1985;92:444–448
9. Avila MP, Jalkh AE, Feldman E, et al. Manifestations of Whipple's disease in the posterior segment of the eye. Arch Ophthalmol 1984;102:384–390
10. Graham EM, Stanford MR, Sanders MD, et al. A point prevalence study of 150 patients with idiopathic retinal vasculitis. I. Diagnostic value of ophthalmological features. Br J Ophthalmol 1986;73:714–721
11. Michelson JB, Chisari FV. Behçet's disease. Surv Ophthalmol 1982;26:190–203
12. Lehner T, Barnes CG, eds. Recent advances in Behçet's disease. London: Royal Society of Medicine Services, 1986
13. Mullaney J, Collum LMT. Ocular vasculitis in Behçet's disease. Int Ophthalmol 1985;7:183–191
14. Rucker CW. Sheathing of the retinal veins in multiple sclerosis. Mayo Clin Proc 1944;19:176–178
15. Lightman S, McDonald WI, Bird AC, et al. Retinal venous sheathing in optic neuritis. Brain 1987;110:405–414
16. Graham EM, Francis DA, Sanders MD, Rudge P. Ocular inflammatory changes in established multiple sclerosis. J Neurol Neurosurg Psychiatry 1989;52:1360–1363
17. Miller DH, Rudge P, Johnson G, et al. Serial Gadolinium enhanced magnetic resonance imaging in multiple sclerosis. Brain 1988;111:927–939
18. Wakefield D, Abi-Hanna D. HLA antigens and their significance in the pathogenesis of anterior uveitis: a mini review. Curr Eye Res 1986;5:465–473
19. Ruby AJ, Jampol LM. Crohn's disease and retinal vascular disease. Am J Ophthalmol 1990;110:349–353
20. Issak BL, Liesegang TJ, Michet CJ. Ocular and systemic findings in relapsing polychondritis. Ophthalmology 1986;93:681–689

Systemic Associations of Pigmentary Retinopathy

Arlene V. Drack, M.D.

Elias I. Traboulsi, M.D.

Pigmentary retinopathy is the final common pathway for many retinal and chorioretinal disorders and one manifestation of many metabolic and neurodegenerative diseases. Pigmentary retinopathy corresponds to hyperplasia and migration of the retinal pigment epithelium into the neurosensory retina, usually along blood vessels. This process is often more prominent in the periphery than in the posterior pole of the retina. Pigmentary retinopathy is a nonspecific sign rather than a diagnosis. For this reason, the evaluation of patients with pigmentary retinopathy is a special challenge. The same fundus picture may represent a primary ocular process, a harbinger of neurological degeneration, a remote effect of cancer [1], or just one feature in a constellation of signs comprising a genetic syndrome.

Ophthalmoscopic findings in typical *retinitis pigmentosa* (RP) include waxy atrophy of the optic nerve head, narrowing of the retinal vessels, and bony spicule clumping of pigment in the retinal periphery (Fig 1). *Atypical RP* refers to a pattern of pigmentary retinopathy that differs from classical RP (as just described) in its pattern of distribution and degree of pigment migration in the fundus. *Retinal dystrophy* is a broad term that includes genetic retinal disease as well as pigmentary and nonpigmentary retinopathies in inherited systemic disorders. We do not use the term *retinal degeneration* in this chapter, although it may be found to be appropriate by other authors.

In the workup of the patient with pigmentary retinopathy, a meticulous history of the onset and course of ocular symptoms should be taken, as well as a complete review of systems with special emphasis on disease processes known to be associated with a retinal dystrophy. A detailed family history is essential, and a general physical examination should be performed in addition to the ocular examination. An electroretinogram (ERG) may be helpful in characterizing pigmentary retinopathies but is rarely diagnostic. Additional biochemical and metabolic tests, neurological imaging, and referral to appropriate specialists in other medical fields must be obtained as needed. The etiology of RP is being unraveled through the recent discovery of point mutations in the rhodopsin gene in some patients with dominant RP [2, 3]. Many

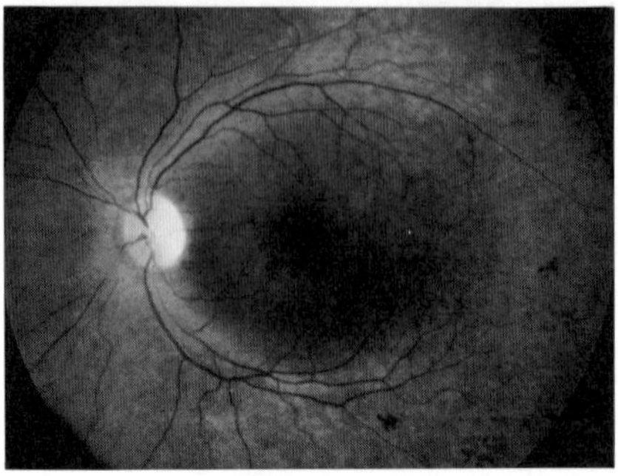

Figure 1 *Ophthalmoscopic appearance in typical retinitis pigmentosa with waxy pallor of the optic nerve head, attenuation of retinal vessels, and peripheral pigmentary changes in a bony spicule configuration.*

other factors, including immune defects [4] and abnormal amino acid [5], vitamin A [6], and lipid [7] metabolism have been thought to play a role in both primary and secondary retinal dystrophies. In secondary pigmentary retinopathies in which an underlying systemic abnormality is known, we have the unique opportunity to study the effect of various metabolic defects on the retina.

This chapter deals with some of the systemic diseases that are associated with pigmentary retinopathy. Some of these diseases inevitably fall into more than one of the categories listed in Table 1 but are discussed under the most inclusive heading.

■ Disorders of Amino Acid, Protein, and Lipoprotein Metabolism

Gyrate Atrophy of Choroid and Retina

Gyrate atrophy of the choroid and retina is an autosomal recessive disorder characterized by progressive myopia, chorioretinal atrophic lesions, peripheral visual field loss, and night blindness starting in the first decade of life [8]. Blindness ensues by age 40 to 50 years in most untreated patients [9]. Mild proximal muscle weakness is clinically demonstrable in a minority of patients, although most show abnormalities in muscle fibers on biopsy [10]. Approximately one-third of patients have slow waves on electroencephalography [11]. Fine, straight, sparse hair may be present [12].

The chorioretinopathy of gyrate atrophy is characteristic. Geographical, round or oval areas of choroidal and retinal atrophy appear in the peripheral fundus; these areas enlarge and coalesce giving an appearance similar to cerebral gyri (Fig 2). Peripapillary lesions may be seen even while the disc remains pink and healthy (Fig 3). The atrophic areas are separated from normal-appearing retina by hyperpigmented areas, and crystals have been reported at the margins of the atrophic areas [13]. Posterior subcapsular cataracts develop by the second or third decade [14]. The ERG is decreased late in the disease but before the atrophy becomes complete. Fluorescein angiography shows hyperfluorescence in affected areas, with staining at the edges of normal-appearing retina. The histopathological features of the eyes of an older patient with the disease have recently been reported by Wilson and co-workers [15].

Table 1 *Systemic Syndromes Associated with Pigmentary Retinopathy*

Disorders of amino acid, protein, and lipoprotein metabolism
Gyrate atrophy of the choroid and retina
Cystinosis
Cobalamin C defects (methylmalonic aciduria with homocystinuria)
Abetalipoproteinemia
Lysosomal storage diseases
Mucopolysaccharidosis IH (Hurler's syndrome)
Mucopolysaccharidosis IS (Scheie's syndrome)
Mucopolysaccharidosis II (Hunter's syndrome)
Mucopolysaccharidosis IIIA and IIIB (Sanfilippo's syndrome)
Mucolipidosis IV
Peroxisomal disorders
Cerebrohepatorenal syndrome (Zellweger's syndrome)
Neonatal adrenoleukodystrophy
Refsum's disease
Neurological and neuromuscular disorders
Neuronal ceroid lipofuscinoses
Olivopontocerebellar atrophy with retinal degeneration (OPCA type III)
Kearns-Sayre syndrome
Myotonic dystrophy
Hallervoden-Spatz syndrome
Joubert's syndrome
Flynn-Aird syndrome
Dermatological disorders
Darier's disease
Renal disease
Retinal-renal dysplasia (Senior-Loken syndrome)
Skeletal anomalies and dwarfism
Asphyxiating thoracic dystrophy (Jeune's syndrome)
Cockayne's syndrome
Bardet-Biedl syndrome
Osteopetrosis
Retinitis pigmentosa and deafness
Usher's syndrome types I and II
Alstrom's syndrome
Miscellaneous disorders
Alagille's syndrome (arteriohepatic dysplasia)
Infectious diseases
Rubella
Syphilis

Gyrate atrophy is caused by a deficiency of the enzyme ornithine aminotransferase (OAT) with resultant hyperornithinemia [12, 16]. The OAT gene has been cloned and analyzed [17]. There is genetic heterogeneity, and the disease may result from a number of point mutations in the OAT gene in some patients and from deletions in others [18–21]. Some patients with gyrate atrophy respond to treatment with pharmacological doses of pyridoxine [22].

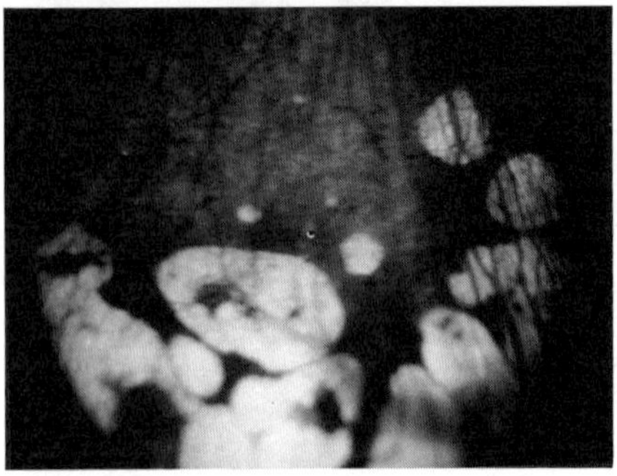

Figure 2 *Fundus of a 9-year-old girl with gyrate atrophy of the choroid and retina. Note confluent areas of atrophy in a gyrate pattern and clumps of pigment in adjacent areas.*

A diet restricted in arginine (a precursor of ornithine) has been shown to bring plasma ornithine levels into the normal range [23] and may halt the progression of the retinopathy in some cases. Proline supplementation has also been reported to slow the retinopathy [24].

Cystinosis

Cystinosis is an autosomal recessive condition characterized by progressive renal failure, retinopathy, growth retardation, and deposition of cystine crystals in many tissues of the body [25]. Hypothyroidism, diabetes mellitus, dysphagia, and neurological changes have also been reported. A lysosomal defect probably prevents the transport of cystine from lysosomes into the cytosol, and crystals form inside lysosomes [26]. Three main clinical types of cystinosis are recognized: The first is an early infantile nephropathic form that presents at 8 to 12 months of age with polydypsia, polyuria, recurrent fever, acidosis, and rickets. Renal failure occurs in the first decade of life. Most patients fall into this first category. The second type is a late-onset form in which renal failure may not ensue until the second or third decade of life, and the third is a benign form in which retinopathy and renal failure do not occur [27].

The ocular findings in cystinosis include crystalline corneal deposits that are best demonstrated on slit-lamp examination and that lead to significant

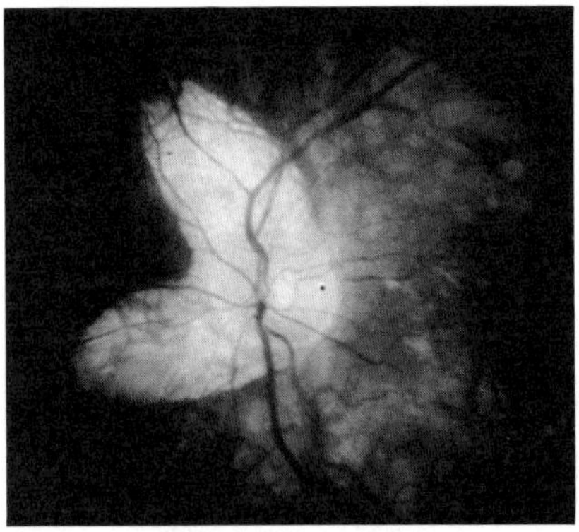

Figure 3 *Peripapillary lesion in fundus of same patient as in Figure 2. Optic papilla was otherwise normal.*

photophobia [28, 29]. Retinal pigmentary changes are typical [30] and appear initially in the fundus periphery but progress to involve the macula. There are mottled areas of depigmentation and pigment clumping with or without yellowish macular changes. Deep retinal crystals may be seen. Retinal changes may precede the appearance of corneal crystals. The retinopathy is more common in the infantile form and was present in all patients with infantile cystinosis by age 7 years in one long-term study [31]. The optic nerve, visual fields, ERG, and electrooculogram (EOG) are generally normal; the ERG may, however, decrease in amplitude with time [31].

Cystinosis is diagnosed by the presence of crystals in biopsy material and by an 80- to 100-fold increase in free cystine in peripheral leukocytes or cultured skin fibroblasts. Prenatal diagnosis may be possible by chorionic villus biopsy. Treatment is necessary to correct the metabolic aberrations, and renal transplantation is usually required in the nephropathic varieties. Systemic administration of cysteamine has been beneficial [32], and cysteamine has also been used topically to improve corneal clarity [33]. Growth hormone [34] and oral carnitine [35] have been used as well.

Methylmalonic Aciduria with Homocystinuria

Methylmalonic aciduria with homocystinuria results from at least three autosomal recessive disorders of cobalamin transport and metabolism [36]. Patients usually present in the first few months of life with failure to thrive, developmental delay, seizures, and megaloblastic anemia. Some patients may present later in childhood with fatigue and neurological symptoms.

Ocular findings include fine pigmentary changes in the retinal periphery and granular or bull's-eye maculopathy [37, 38]. Nystagmus, optic nerve pallor, attenuated retinal vessels, and strabismus can occur. The ERG is attenuated early in the course of the disease.

Methylmalonic aciduria with homocystinuria is due to abnormal cobalamin metabolism (possibly a defect of cytosolic cobalamin reductase), which leads to deficient activity of L-methylmalonyl coenzyme A mutase and N-methyltetrahydrofolate:homocysteine methyltransferase. This, in turn, leads to elevated levels of homocysteine with methylmalonic acid in the urine and low levels of blood methionine. In one patient, there was a failure of release of free vitamin B_{12} from lysosomes [39].

Early treatment with very large doses (up to 1 mg/day intramuscularly) of hydroxycobalamin with or without betaine improves the biochemical profiles, and possibly the outcome, of some patients [40]. There is evidence that metronidazole may be helpful in reducing gut flora that produce propionic acid, which in turn is metabolized to methylmalonic acid [41].

Abetalipoproteinemia

Abetalipoproteinemia (Bassen-Kornzweig disease) is a rare autosomal recessive disorder [42] initially described in Ashkenazi Jews. Subsequent cases have been reported in other ethnic groups as well [43]. Systemic findings include acanthocytosis, mild fat malabsorption and steatorrhea, progressive spinocerebellar degeneration, and abnormal plasma lipids with total absence of lipoproteins and chylomicra. All major plasma lipids are reduced to less than 50% of normal levels. The deficiency in chylomicra prevents absorption of fat-soluble vitamins from the intestine, leading to low serum levels of vitamins A and E [44, 45]. The underlying defect is believed to be abnormal production of beta-protein-containing lipoproteins by liver and intestinal cells [46]. The main ocular manifestation of abetalipoproteinemia is an atypical pigmentary retinopathy that develops in the early teens but can present at any age. The fundus findings are similar to RP in some cases and to retinitis punctata albescens in others [47, 48]. The ERG demonstrates rod and cone dysfunction, and dark adaptation thresholds may be elevated before ophthalmoscopic changes appear [49]. The macula may or may not be affected. Angioid streaks have also been described.

The low levels of serum fat-soluble vitamins may account for the pigmentary retinopathy. Hypovitaminosis E [45] and A [47] have been suspected to be causal. There is evidence that oral vitamin E therapy improves the neuropathy and slows or prevents the retinopathy [45, 50]. Vitamin A supplementation has been reported to have beneficial retinal effects as well [48].

■ Lysosomal Storage Diseases

Mucopolysaccharidoses

Mucopolysaccharidosis IH (MPS-IH), also known as Hurler's syndrome, is an autosomal recessive disorder in which there is progressive accumulation of acid mucopolysaccharides in body tissues due to deficiency of alpha-L-iduronidase [51]. This leads to coarse facies with thick lips and enlarged tongue. Developmental delay, hepatosplenomegaly, and dwarfism are apparent by 1 to 3 years of age. Joint contractures and kyphoscoliosis develop, and roentgenograms show what has been termed *dysostosis multiplex.* Ocular findings include corneal clouding and a rod-cone dystrophy. Photophobia and night blindness may be early symptoms. The retinal pigmentary changes may be subtle, with an abnormal ERG [52]. Papilledema may be seen and is possibly due to optic nerve compression at the lamina cribrosa secondary to posterior scleral thickening with mucopolysaccharides [53]. Glaucoma has been reported in a few cases. Although the exact cause of the retinopathy is unknown, only those mucopolysaccharidoses in which heparan sulfate is stored are associated with a retinal dystrophy. Ocular histopathological findings have been reported in a few cases [54, 55].

Most patients with MPS-IH die by 10 years of age from respiratory or cardiac causes. Bone marrow transplantation trials are under way. Visual success following corneal grafting may be compromised by retinal or optic nerve pathological processes.

MPS-IS (Scheie's syndrome) has laboratory findings identical to those in MPS-IH. The difference between the two diseases is one of severity of clinical findings: Hepatosplenomegaly, mental retardation, and dwarfism do not occur in MPS-IS. Facial features are less dysmorphic. Corneal clouding and retinal dystrophy are present, however, with resultant decreased vision. Deafness, genu valgum, and joint stiffness develop. Aortic regurgitation and psychosis are occasional findings [51].

Diagnostic techniques are the same as in MPS-IH, but supportive treatment may be more successful. Patients generally live to adulthood.

MPS-III (Sanfilippo's syndrome) is an autosomal recessive storage disease in which heparitin sulfate is excreted in the urine due to a deficiency in one of four enzymes that degrade acid mucopolysaccharides. Like MPS-IH and MPS-IS, the accumulation of mucopolysaccharides is generalized, but in MPS-III the somatic stigmata are mild, whereas the severe central nervous system consequences are devastating. Four distinct enzymatic defects can be detected in fibroblasts, but the clinical picture is the same. Patients are normal in appearance and development in infancy. Motor delay, intellectual deterioration, and behavioral problems become apparent by school age. There is rapid clinical deterioration and, if patients live to adulthood, they are bedridden and demented. Deafness may also develop.

Corneal clouding is not a feature of MPS-III, but a pigmentary retinopathy similar to MPS-IH and MPS-IS is present. Ocular histopathological findings in type IIIA have been reported by Del Monte and colleagues [56] and in type IIIB by Lavery and co-workers [57].

The appearance of bony spicules in the retina, often with optic atrophy and chronic papilledema, is also seen in MPS-II (Hunter's syndrome) [52]. The cornea is clear. Systemic features include coarse facies, stiff joints, and dwarfism. In MPS-IIA, life span is shortened and mental retardation is present. In MPS-IIB, life span and intellect may be normal. Both types are caused by a defect in iduronate sulfatase. Inheritance is X-linked recessive.

Mucolipidosis IV

Mucolipidosis IV, a recessive disorder, is characterized by normal development in the first few months of life followed by psychomotor retardation, corneal clouding, retinal dystrophy, athetosis, and progressive motor and mental disability. There are no skeletal or visceral abnormalities [58]. Corneal clouding quickly prevents visualization of the fundus. When the corneal epithelium is removed, optic atrophy and retinal dystrophy become apparent. The ocular histopathology was studied by Riedel and co-workers [59]. Although the disease was originally described in Ashkenazi Jews, it has also been reported in non-Jewish families.

Deficiency of ganglioside sialidase in mucolipidosis IV [60] has recently been refuted [61]. Diagnosis is based on clinical findings and on the demonstration of characteristic intracellular inclusions in conjunctival biopsies [62]. Corneal clarity can be achieved temporarily by removal of the corneal epithelium and by conjunctival transplantation using donor tissue from unaffected siblings [63]. Patients may survive into early adulthood but are profoundly retarded [58].

■ Peroxisomal Disorders

The peroxisomopathies are a heterogeneous group of disorders in which there is dysfunction or absence of peroxisomes or absence of peroxisomal enzymes that are involved in a number of oxidative and other cellular reactions

Table 2 *Classification of Human Peroxisomal Disorders*

Group 1: Peroxisomes are lacking; multiple enzymatic defects
Zellweger's syndrome
Neonatal adrenoleukodystrophy
Hyperpipecolic acidemia
Infantile phytanic acid storage disease
Group 2: Intact peroxisomal structure; more than one enzymatic defect
Rhizomelic chondrodysplasia punctata
Group 3: Intact peroxisomal structure; single enzymatic defect
X-linked childhood adrenoleukodystrophy
Hyperoxaluria type I
Acyl-coenzyme A oxidase deficiency
Pseudo-Zellweger's syndrome
Acatalasemia
Adult Refsum's disease

Source: Modified from Moser HW, Peroxisomal disorders. J Pediatr 1986; 108:89–91.

[64, 65]. The biochemical hallmark of several of the peroxisomal disorders is elevation of very long chain fatty acids, pipecolic acid, and decreased levels of plasmalogens. Patients with some peroxisomopathies have an infantile type of retinal dystrophy that mimics Leber's congenital amaurosis, and such patients were indeed misdiagnosed as having the latter condition before peroxisomopathies were recognized [66]. Moser [67] classifies the peroxisomopathies into three main groups (Table 2).

Zellweger's Syndrome

Zellweger's syndrome is the prototype of peroxisomal diseases and is characterized by infantile hypotonia, psychomotor retardation, seizures, a characteristic facies, renal cortical cysts, and hepatic interstitial fibrosis [68]. Inheritance is autosomal recessive. Most patients die before 1 year of age.

Ocular findings include nystagmus, cloudy cornea, congenital glaucoma, cataract, retinal dystrophy and, occasionally, optic nerve hypoplasia [69]. The ERG is moderately to severely decreased in amplitude. Ocular histopathological evaluation reveals photoreceptor dropout and loss of ganglion cells along with a variety of anterior segment malformations [70].

Neonatal Adrenoleukodystrophy

Patients with neonatal adrenoleukodystrophy present with hypotonia, seizures, and psychomotor retardation in infancy [71]. Death occurs by 7 years of age. Adrenal atrophy is seen on autopsy. Ocular findings include decreased vision with nystagmus, cataracts, and a pigmentary retinopathy with optic atrophy. The ocular histopathological findings have been studied by Cohen and co-workers [72] and Glasgow and associates [73].

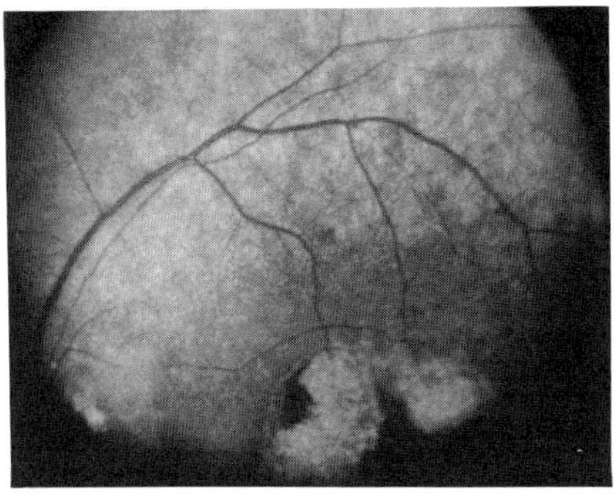

Figure 4 *Left fundus of 30-year-old man with Refsum's disease showing mild fine pigmentary changes, atrophy of the retinal pigment epithelium, narrowing of the retinal arterioles, and a macular atrophic scar. (Courtesy of Irene H. Maumenee, M.D.)*

Refsum's Disease

Refsum's disease (phytanic acid storage disease) is an autosomal recessive condition characterized by cerebellar ataxia, polyneuropathy, pigmentary retinopathy, anosmia, deafness, ichthyosis, and cardiac myopathy with arrhythmias [74]. Cerebrospinal fluid protein concentration is increased without pleocytosis. Symptoms may be present in childhood, but diagnosis is often not made until adulthood.

Night blindness may be an early symptom. Ophthalmoscopy reveals a progressive pigmentary retinopathy with atrophic macular lesions in some patients (personal observation, 1985) (Fig 4). In other patients, the fundus picture is similar to typical RP [75]. Central visual function is preserved early in the course of the disease, but severe visual impairment eventually develops. Ptosis and ophthalmoplegia have been reported and make differentiation from Kearns-Sayre syndrome and from advanced olivopontocerebellar atrophy with retinal degeneration (vide infra) essential.

Diagnosis is made by demonstration of elevated plasma levels of phytanic acid. In some patients, phytanic acid levels are normal, and assay for phytanic acid oxidase activity should be obtained. Acute treatment with plasmapheresis may be beneficial. Dietary restriction of phytanic acid can prevent many of the disease sequelae, but the retinal dystrophy and deafness may continue to progress.

Infantile Phytanic Acid Storage Disease

Infantile phytanic acid storage disease has its onset in the first few years of life and is characterized by dysmorphic facies, mental retardation, hepatomegaly, and retinal dystrophy [76]. Serum levels of phytanic acid are elevated. Affected infants have poor vision and nystagmus with a pigmentary retinopathy, optic nerve pallor, macular atrophic changes, and arteriolar narrowing. Fluorescein angiography shows diffuse retinal pigment epithelium (RPE) and choriocapillaris dropout, and the ERG shows decreased rod and cone responses [77].

Neurological and Neuromuscular Disorders

Neuronal Ceroid Lipofuscinoses

The neuronal ceroid lipofuscinoses (NCLs) comprise a group of autosomal recessive disorders characterized by progressive neurological deterioration, seizures, and pigmentary retinopathy with progressive visual loss in early-onset cases. Four types are described: infantile (Haltia-Santavuori syndrome) with onset at 8 to 18 months of age; late infantile (Jansky-Bielschowsky syndrome) with onset between 2 and 4 years old; juvenile (Vogt-Spielmeyer-Batten syndrome) with onset at 4 to 8 years old, and adult-onset (Kufs' syndrome) [78–81]. In the infantile and late infantile forms, neurological degeneration usually precedes retinopathy and vision loss; in the adult form, no ophthalmological manifestations are present. Therefore, it is patients with juvenile NCL who present first to the ophthalmologist with complaints of decreased vision. The infantile form of NCL may initially present like Rett's syndrome with hand stereotypy, and the ophthalmologist may be able to make the correct diagnosis if characteristic NCL retinal dystrophy develops later [82]. The gene for the infantile form of NCL has been mapped to chromosome 1 [83].

The systemic manifestations of the NCLs include dementia, behavioral changes, psychomotor deterioration, ataxia, and seizures. There is abnormal accumulation of autofluorescent retinoidlike substances, ceroid, lipofuscin, phospholipids, free fatty acids, and cholesterol esters [78–80]. The underlying defect may be an abnormality in the dolichol pathway or a deficiency in free-radical protective mechanisms. It is not known how the accumulation of these substances causes the neurological and retinal damage. Antioxidant therapy trials have not been effective.

Ocular findings in infantile NCL include optic atrophy, macular pigmentary changes with mottling of the retinal periphery, and low or absent ERG amplitude and low visual evoked responses (VER) [84]; cataracts have also been reported [81]. In the late infantile form, there is a bull's-eye maculopathy, pigment mottling and granularity, optic atrophy, and attenuation of retinal blood vessels. The juvenile form shows an absent macular reflex and, at times, a bull's-eye maculopathy (Fig 5); there are also peripheral RPE changes, optic atrophy, and attenuation of the retinal blood vessels [80]. There are no clinical

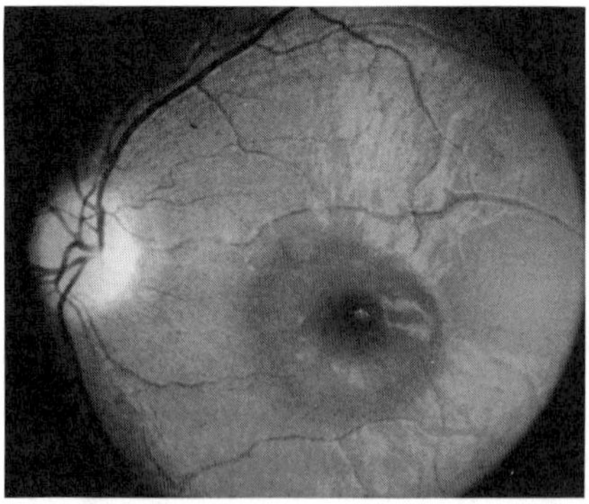

Figure 5 *Left fundus of a 7-year-old girl with late infantile neuronal ceroid lipofuscinosis showing bull's-eye maculopathy.*

ocular findings in the adult form of NCL, although retinal storage has been demonstrated [85].

Diagnosis can be made by history and clinical findings, the presence of consanguinity, and the demonstration of typical curvilinear and fingerprint inclusions on electron microscopy in different body tissues including conjunctiva, skin, lymphocytes [86], and rectal mucosa. Prenatal diagnosis is possible by demonstrating the diagnostic cellular inclusions in amniocytes or chorionic villi [87, 88].

Olivopontocerebellar Atrophy with Retinal Degeneration

Olivopontocerebellar atrophy (OPCA) is the major radiological feature of a heterogeneous group of neurodegenerative disorders [89]. Only one type (type III in the classification of Koenigsmark and Weiner [90]) is associated with retinal degeneration. Inheritance is autosomal dominant, but the age of onset varies widely, even within a single family [91, 92]. When the disease presents in infancy, there is developmental delay, ataxia, and poor vision. Seizures are uncommon. There is diffuse pigmentary mottling of the retina, with a diminished ERG. Strabismus may be present. Death occurs in the first few years of life. When the disease presents in childhood or adolescence, it proceeds at a slower rate with progressive cerebellar ataxia, dysarthria, and blindness. Adult-onset disease has an even more slowly progressive course, with gradually increasing ataxia and decreased vision. Visual loss with predominant macular involvement may be the presenting findings in older patients, with progression to diffuse pigmentary retinopathy and peripheral punched-out chorioretinal lesions resembling gyrate atrophy (personal observations) and severe loss of vision [92–94]. Subtle cerebellar signs should be sought. Ophthalmoplegia may develop gradually. Ocular pathological findings in infants and adults reveal photoreceptor dropout with sparing of the ganglion cells and optic nerve, which is mirrored clinically [92, 95]. In the brain, there is Purkinje cell dropout.

Diagnosis is based on clinical findings unless pathological findings are obtained in a family member. Neuroimaging reveals pontine and cerebellar atrophy. OPCA type III should be suspected in infants presenting with a neurodegenerative disease and retinal dystrophy and should be differentiated from infantile phytanic acid storage disease, abetalipoproteinemia, recessive neonatal adrenoleukodystrophy, and the infantile form of NCL. One parent is frequently mildly affected in OPCA type III, and the dominant mode of inheritance along with the clinical presence of ataxia are the best differential diagnostic clues. The family history may not be helpful in cases where the affected parent has not yet developed the disease at the time when the child is symptomatic. Epilepsy and microcephaly are frequently seen in infantile NCL and are absent in OPCA type III.

Kearns-Sayre Syndrome

The three major components of the Kearns-Sayre syndrome (KSS) are ophthalmoplegia, an atypical pigmentary retinopathy, and cardiac conduction defects [96]. Additional clinical findings include cerebellar ataxia, proximal muscle weakness, hearing loss, and vestibular dysfunction. Endocrinological abnormalities in some patients include hypothyroidism and hypoparathyroidism. There may be increased levels of cerebrospinal fluid protein. Serum creatine kinase is normal. Complete and incomplete forms of the disease have been recognized, with variation in the number of systems involved, severity, and age of onset of clinical disease.

The ocular findings in KSS include a progressive external ophthalmoplegia with ptosis, starting in the second decade of life, and an atypical pigmentary retinopathy with hypopigmentation and hyperpigmentation of the RPE with or without ERG abnormalities and usually without severe visual dysfunction. This is most marked in the macular and peripapillary zones [97, 98]. Earlier onset of visual symptoms seems to correlate with a poorer visual outcome. Significant pigmentary changes in the fundus may not be accompanied by reduction in the ERG potential or by decreased visual acuity. The course of the retinopathy is usually one of slow progression with maintenance of good visual function until late in life in most patients.

Histological, structural, and functional defects of mitochondria have been identified in KSS. Ragged red fibers are present on histological sections of muscle tissue [99]. Deletions of mitochondrial DNA were present in 32 of 123 patients with mitochondrial myopathies, including 15 patients with KSS and 17 patients with ocular myopathy, but not in other mitochondrial encephalomyopathies [100]. This reinforces the view that KSS is a specific disorder among the mitochondrial encephalomyopathies. The presence of these mitochondrial DNA deletions in progressive external ophthalmoplegia without other features of KSS suggests that KSS is the full expression of a pleiotropic disorder. The predominant affection of the extraocular muscles may be due to their high content of mitochondria (the mitochondrial volume of extraocular muscles is three to four times that of limb muscles) or because of mitotic segregations in the zygote resulting in uneven distribution of mitochondrial genomes in different tissues. The majority of patients with KSS are isolated cases with no family history of the disease; however, the genetic nature of the disease is evident because of the DNA deletions and the few reports of familial occurrences [101–103]. The mitochondrial DNA deletions have also been identified in several tissues including muscle, blood, liver, brain, and skin.

Myotonic Dystrophy

Myotonic dystrophy is an autosomal dominant disorder with variable penetrance. In patients with late-onset disease, weakness and atrophy of many muscle groups, including the face and extremities, occurs. Patients have characteristic facies with hollow cheeks and sagging jaws. Cardiac conduction defects are present in the majority of patients but are seldom lethal. Testicular atrophy is present in approximately 80% of men with the disease. Other findings include frontal balding in men, hypoventilation, disturbances in swallowing and gastrointestinal motility, club feet in approximately 50% of cases, behavioral changes, and central nervous system abnormalities. Basal metabolic rates are low, and there is hyperinsulinemia but no diabetes mellitus. Myotonia may not be symptomatic but can be elicited by asking the patient to grasp something and release the grip quickly (release and relaxation will be delayed) or by percussing the thenar area and demonstrating prolonged muscular contraction. Congenital cases occur only in children born to affected mothers. Surprisingly, this is not transient as in myasthenia gravis, and all these infants progress to become affected adults with myotonia developing by 3 years of age. The precise etiology of the associated anomalies is unknown, but muscle excitability may be altered by circulating factors or membrane abnormalities. Genetic linkage to chromosome 19q markers has been demonstrated [104]. Very few cases of myotonic dystrophy are due to new mutations, and affected family members with mild manifestations of the disease should be identified.

Ocular findings are not present in childhood. In older patients, a progressive macular or peripheral pigmentary retinopathy develops unaccompanied by visual loss [105, 106]. ERG shows decreased photopic and scotopic b waves with delayed scotopic implicit time [106]. Iridescent lenticular opacities (Christmas-tree cataract) are almost always present and are characteristic [107]. Mild ptosis is common, and there may be limitation to ocular movements with normal forced duction tests. Ocular hypotony is present in one-third of patients [108].

Treatment is supportive. There is an increased risk of malignant hyperthermia, and appropriate precautions should be taken prior to and during surgical procedures.

Hallervorden-Spatz Syndrome

Hallervorden-Spatz syndrome is a recessive condition with progressive rigidity of the extremities, extrapyramidal motor signs, dysarthria, dementia and, ultimately, death [109]. Because early symptoms are insidious and unusual, psychological disorders may be suspected, but coexistent depression may be a feature of the disorder [110]. The hallmark of this condition is the deposition of iron, most notably in the globus pallidus and the substantia nigra [111, 112]. Diagnosis is made on clinical and neuroradiological grounds. A distinctive feature of Hallervorden-Spatz syndrome is neuroaxonal degeneration with formation of spheroid bodies or inclusions [113]. Acanthocytosis is present in some patients [114, 115]. Almost 25% of patients have retinal degeneration [109]. Such individuals are young and have rapidly progressive disease. There is a flecked type of retinopathy with bull's-eye maculopathy; typical RP-like changes develop later. Ocular histopathological findings have been reported by Luckenback and colleagues [113] and by Roth and associates [116].

Joubert's Syndrome

Joubert's syndrome is an autosomal recessive disorder in which infantile respiratory difficulties (hyperpnea, apnea) and developmental delay are associated with decreased vision and a retinal picture identical to that of Leber's congenital amaurosis [117]. A pigmentary retinopathy develops with a normal VER and an abnormal ERG [118]. An ocular motility disorder similar to oculomotor apraxia, and nystagmus may be present. Neuroimaging studies reveal hypoplasia of the cerebellar vermis.

Flynn-Aird Syndrome

Flynn-Aird syndrome is a rare autosomal dominant syndrome combining deafness, neurological degeneration with atypical seizures, and skin and bone defects. Deafness is usually the presenting sign, developing in early adulthood. Ataxia, neuritic pain, atrophic skin lesions, and joint stiffness follow. The underlying defect is unknown. Ocular findings include high myopia, cataracts, and RP [119].

■ Dermatological Disorders

Darier's disease is a rare autosomal dominant disorder with variable expressivity. The skin manifestations of Darier's disease include a follicular keratosis with papules, scaly crust, and papillomatous masses. Nails are dystrophic, and there may be pitting of the palms. Two brothers with the disease were reported by Itin and co-workers [120] to have typical RP with bone spicules in the retina, progressive visual field loss to 5 to 10 degrees, narrowed retinal arterioles, and pale discs. Cataracts were present in both brothers at an early age. The ERG was extinguished at the ages of 48 and 52 years. Deficient dark adaptation without typical retinal findings has been described in other patients with Darier's disease [121]. Vitamin A therapy usually improves the skin lesions of Darier's disease, though it has not been shown to improve RP.

■ Renal Disease

Senior-Loken syndrome (nephronophthisis-retinopathy syndrome, retinal-renal dysplasia) is an autosomal recessive condition in which medullary cystic kidney disease secondary to a chronic, nondestructive, interstitial nephritis leads to renal failure in the first decade of life [122, 123]. The ocular findings may be of two types. In the first type, children present in the first year of life with blindness and have a retinal picture identical to that in Leber's congenital amaurosis. The ERG response is absent, there is nystagmus, and the retina may appear normal or show areas of hypopigmentation and hyperpigmentation with arteriolar narrowing [124–126]. In the second type, the onset of retinal dystrophy occurs later in life [127]. Because the ophthalmologist may make the diagnosis of Leber's congenital amaurosis long before renal failure occurs, all such patients should have serial tests of renal function and should be counseled about the possibility of having this disease. There are also reports of liver fibrosis and mental retardation, but these may represent patients with Zellweger's syndrome [128, 129]. A single recessive gene may be responsible for both the ocular and renal disorders [130].

■ Skeletal Anomalies

Asphyxiating Thoracic Dystrophy

Asphyxiating thoracic dystrophy (Jeune's syndrome) is an autosomal recessive disorder characterized by variable degrees of short-limbed dwarfism, thoracic dysplasia with respiratory insufficiency, brachydactyly and, in some cases, polydactyly, with cone-shaped epiphyses, liver abnormalities, and progressive renal failure. The underlying genetic or metabolic defect is not known. Respiratory insufficiency frequently results in death in infancy, but some patients survive to adulthood. Ocular findings consist of midperipheral and, at times, macular RPE disturbance [131]. Visual acuity may be reduced, and myopia, photophobia, nystagmus, and strabismus have been described. ERG and visual field defects are progressive [132]. Histopathological study of the retina of one patient showed mild changes of the RPE, marked loss of photoreceptor cells with relative sparing of cones, and moderate loss of peripheral ganglion cells [133].

Cockayne's Syndrome

Cockayne's syndrome is a rare autosomal recessive disorder in which patients exhibit dwarfism, progeria, deafness, mental retardation, skin photosensitivity, and birdlike facies [134]. Development may be normal in the first year of life, with deterioration thereafter. Death usually occurs before the teenage years, with occasional survival into the third decade. There may be a defect in the ability of cells to repair ultraviolet-induced DNA damage [135].

Ocular findings include enophthalmos, which is universal and is due to loss of subcutaneous and orbital fat, poor pupillary dilation due to hypoplasia of the dilator muscle with iris transillumination, and cataracts that develop in the second decade of life [136, 137]. There is an atypical pigmentary retinopathy characterized by fine granular pigment spots, attenuated retinal vessels, and optic atrophy. Heavier scattered black pigmentation may be more pronounced in the posterior pole. There is no tendency to typical bone spicule formation. The ERG response is decreased or extinguished. High hyperopic and astigmatic refractive errors are universal. Corneal dystrophic changes and recurrent erosions have been described in several patients and usually involve the lower half of the cornea [138]. Photophobia may be extreme.

Diagnosis may be aided by magnetic resonance imaging of the brain, which may show hypomyelination, cerebellar atrophy, and calcification of the basal ganglia. Ultraviolet irradiation of cultured fibroblasts results in abnormal DNA repair. The differential diagnosis of Cockayne's syndrome includes Bloom's syndrome, Rothmund-Thomson syndrome, xeroderma pigmentosum, Werner's syndrome, and progeria.

Bardet-Biedl Syndrome

Bardet-Biedl syndrome is an autosomal recessive syndrome that has features evident at birth but may not be diagnosed until later in life. Patients are obese and have postaxial polydactyly (Fig 6), hypogenitalism, hypogonadism, mental retardation, and renal anomalies leading to renal insufficiency and hypertension [139–141]. Diabetes mellitus or glucose intolerance occurs in approximately one-third of patients [142]. The disease is extremely common among the Bedouin in Kuwait [143]. *Laurence-Moon syndrome* is an eponym given to a disorder that is probably identical to the Bardet-Biedl syndrome except for the absence of polydactyly and the presence of spastic paraplegia. A number of other syndromes overlap with the Bardet-Biedl syndrome, and

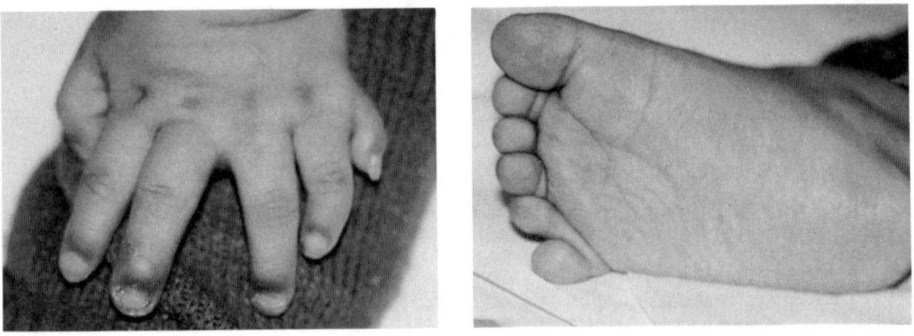

A B

Figure 6 *Postaxial polydactyly in hand (A) and foot (B) of a 4-year-old boy with Bardet-Biedl syndrome.*

it is not clear whether they are genetically distinct or whether they represent variations in the manifestations of the same genetic disease [144]. A progressive retinal dystrophy begins in childhood and progresses to severe visual loss and constriction of visual fields within a few years [145]. Macular pigmentary changes (Fig 7), sometimes in a bull's-eye configuration, and an atypical pigmentary retinopathy develop. Optic nerve pallor and arteriolar narrowing occur, but peripheral pigmentary changes may not be very conspicuous. The ERG is extinguished as in other rod-cone dystrophies [146].

Osteopetrosis

In osteopetrosis, in which deafness and optic atrophy occur secondary to a generalized thickening of calvarial bones that narrow foramina transmitting cranial nerves, a retinal dystrophy has also been reported [147]. Bone marrow transplantation is being tried as a treatment.

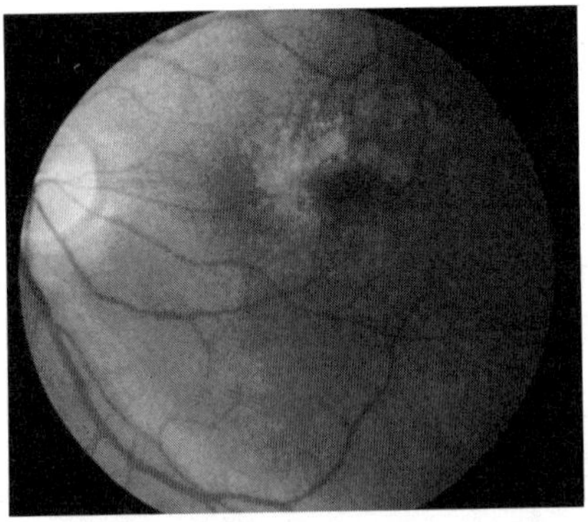

Figure 7 *Macular atrophic changes in a 7-year-old boy with the Bardet-Biedl syndrome. Electroretinographic responses were severely reduced. (Courtesy of Felipe Escallon, MD.)*

Retinitis Pigmentosa and Deafness

Usher's Syndrome

Usher's syndrome is an autosomal recessive condition in which severe sensorineural congenital hearing loss is present in association with RP. Usher's syndrome is the most common cause of deaf-blindness in the United States. At least two types are recognized [148]. In type I, a severe hearing deficit is present from birth and speech rarely develops; vestibular responses are abnormal, and the ERG response is markedly diminished or absent. Ataxia, psychosis, and mental retardation may develop [149]. In type II, hearing loss is less severe; speech may develop, and vestibular and neurological functions are normal. The ERG wave is usually decreased but is recordable. The two types appear to be genetically distinct; the locus for type II has been mapped to chromosome 1q, whereas there is no linkage with type I at this site [150].

Night blindness starts in childhood or the early teen years in type I and later in type II. Central visual acuity is often decreased in the thirties and forties in type I, whereas it may remain at acceptable levels until the fifties or sixties in type II [151]. Ophthalmoscopy reveals findings of typical RP.

Diagnosis is made on the basis of combined otological and ophthalmological testing after other causes of combined RP and deafness have been ruled out. There have been conflicting reports about the frequency of central nervous system abnormalities on neuroimaging [152]. Hunter and co-workers [153] described abnormal axonemes on electron microscopy of sperm and photoreceptors in Usher's syndrome.

Deafness is also seen in association with pigmentary retinopathy in a number of storage diseases, in congenital rubella, Cockayne's syndrome, and Refsum's disease [154].

Alstrom's Syndrome

Alstrom's syndrome includes diabetes mellitus, obesity, and sensorineural deafness with pigmentary retinopathy [155]. Patients may resemble those with Bardet-Biedl syndrome, but there is no polydactyly, and intellect and stature are normal. Presentation is in childhood with decreased vision; progressive decrease in hearing occurs shortly thereafter. Renal disease also develops with age and is often the cause of death. Hypogenitalism is common. Inheritance is autosomal recessive. The pathogenesis of the disease manifestations is unknown.

Ophthalmological findings include retinitis with decreased vision, often before 1 year of age. Salt and pepper retinal pigmentary changes are seen along with areas of atrophy and RPE clumping [156]. The ocular histopathological findings have been reported by Sebag and co-workers [157]. Optic atrophy and arteriolar attenuation are present. Functional blindness by adolescence is usual. Cataracts may be present in some patients.

Miscellaneous Disorders

Alagille's syndrome (arteriohepatic dysplasia) is a disorder characterized by neonatal jaundice secondary to congenital hypoplasia of interlobular bile ducts, with other systemic findings such as dysmorphic facies, pulmonic stenosis, and vertebral and renal anomalies [158]. Inheritance is autosomal dominant with variable penetrance. A deletion of the short arm of chromosome 20 is the probable cause [159]. Patients present in infancy or childhood with jaundice and failure to thrive. Several cases of skin photosensitivity have been reported, with blistering and scarring similar to porphyria. Serum levels of vitamins A and E may be low, and serum porphyrins may be high. Long-term prognosis for liver function is fairly good, though some patients require liver transplants.

The ocular findings include a pigmentary retinopathy with a diminished ERG consistent with rod-cone dystrophy [160]. This may be secondary to low levels of the fat-soluble vitamins, as has been suggested in other disorders. Posterior embryotoxon and other manifestations of anterior segment dysgenesis are common [160]. Keratoconus has been reported in 2 cases [161]. The ocular pathological features have been reported by Johnson [162].

Diagnosis can be made on the basis of clinical, laboratory, or liver biopsy findings. Oral supplementation of vitamins A and E and triglycerides should be considered.

■ Infectious Diseases

Infectious causes of pigmentary retinopathy are many and varied. Intrauterine exposure to infectious agents that cross the placenta can cause a permanent diffuse pigmentary retinopathy as is seen in *congenital rubella* [163]. The congenital rubella syndrome can consist of any combination of pigmentary retinopathy, congenital cataracts, deafness, microphthalmos, microcephaly, and mental retardation. Associated findings that develop later in life include subfoveal neovascular membranes, diabetes mellitus, and thyroid disorders. The pigmentary retinopathy is not, in itself, usually a cause of decreased vision.

Syphilis can cause either a congenital or an acquired pigmentary retinopathy [164]. In congenital syphilis, this may take the form of peripheral pigment mottling or a more typical RP picture. It may be associated with deafness, peglike teeth, keratitis, or rhinitis. The combination of ectopia lentis and pigmentary retinopathy is extremely suggestive of syphilitic oculopathy. In both congenital cases and adults with acquired syphilis, uveitis may be present. A suggestive history should prompt a serological investigation since systemic antibiotics are necessary for treatment.

This work was supported in part by the Krieble and Walter Edel Funds of The Johns Hopkins Center for Hereditary Eye Diseases of The Wilmer Ophthalmological Institute, Baltimore, MD.

■ References

1. van der Pol BA, Planten JT. A non-metastatic remote effect of lung carcinoma. Doc Ophthalmol 1987;67:89–94
2. Dryja TP, McGee TL, Reichel E, et al. A point mutation of the rhodopsin gene in one form of retinitis pigmentosa. Nature 1990;343:364–366

3. Dryja TP, McGee TL, Hahn LB, et al. Mutations within the rhodopsin gene in patients with autosomal dominant retinitis pigmentosa. N Engl J Med 1990; 323:1302–1307
4. Newsome DA, Quinn TC, Hess AD, et al. Cellular immune status in retinitis pigmentosa. Ophthalmology 1988;95:1696–1703
5. Benini G, Marconcini C, Wirth A, et al. Is taurine a marker for retinitis pigmentosa? Ophthalmologica 1988;197:130–135
6. Campbell DA, Tonks EL. Biochemical findings in human retinitis pigmentosa with particular reference to vitamin A deficiency. Br J Ophthalmol 1962;42:151–164
7. Converse CA, Keegan WA, Hug L, et al. Further epidemiologic studies on lipid metabolism in retinitis pigmentosa. Prog Clin Biol Res 1989;314:39–47
8. Kaiser-Kupfer MI, Ludwig IH, DeMonasteris FM, et al. Gyrate atrophy of the choroid and retina: early findings. Ophthalmology 1985;92:394
9. Takki K, Milton RC. The natural history of gyrate atrophy of the choroid and retina. Ophthalmology 1981;88:292
10. Sipila I, Simell O, Rapola J, et al. Gyrate atrophy of the choroid and retina with hyperornithinemia. Tubular aggregates and type 2 fiber atrophy in muscle. Neurology (NY) 1979;29:996–1005
11. Takki K. Gyrate atrophy of the choroid and retina associated with hyperornithinaemia. Br J Ophthalmol 1974;58:3–23
12. Simell O, Takki K. Raised plasma ornithine and gyrate atrophy of the choroid and retina. Lancet 1973;1:1031–1033
13. Kaiser-Kupfer MI, Kuwabara T, Askanas V, et al. Systemic manifestations of gyrate atrophy of the choroid and retina. Ophthalmology 1981;88:302–306
14. Kaiser-Kupfer MI, Kuwabara T, Uga S, et al. Cataracts in gyrate atrophy: clinical and morphologic studies. Invest Ophthalmol Vis Sci 1983;24:432
15. Wilson DJ, Weleber RG, Green WR. Ocular clinicopathologic study of gyrate atrophy. Am J Ophthalmol 1991;111:24–33
16. Kennaway NG, Weleber RG, Buist NRM. Gyrate atrophy of the choroid and retina. Deficient activity of ornithine ketoacid aminotransferase in cultured skin fibroblasts. N Engl J Med 1977;297:1180
17. Mitchell GA, Looney DE, Brody LC, et al. Human ornithine-delta-amino transferase: CDNA cloning and analysis of the structural gene. J Biol Chem 1988; 263:14288
18. Ramesh V, Shaffer MM, Allaire RM, et al. Investigation of gyrate atrophy using a CDNA clone for human ornithine amino transferase. DNA 1986;5:493
19. Inana G, Chambers C, Hatta Y, et al. Point mutation affecting processing of the ornithine aminotransferase precursor protein in gyrate atrophy. J Biol Chem 1989;264:17432–17436
20. Mitchell GM, Brody LC, Looney J, et al. An initiator codon mutation in ornithine-delta-aminotransferase causing gyrate atrophy. J Clin Invest 1988;81:630
21. Inana G, Totsuka S, Fritz C, et al. Expression defect of ornithine-aminotransferase gene in gyrate atrophy. J Clin Invest 1988;29:1001
22. Weleber RG, Kennaway NG, Buist NRM. Vitamin B6 in the management of gyrate atrophy of the choroid and retina. Lancet 1978;2:1213
23. Valle D, Walser M, Brusilow SW, Kaiser-Kupfer M. Gyrate atrophy of the choroid and retina. Amino acid metabolism and correction of hyperornithinemia with an arginine-deficient diet. J Clin Invest 1980;65:371–378
24. Tada K, Saito T, Hayasaka S, et al. Hyperornithinemia with gyrate atrophy: pathophysiology and treatment. J Inherit Metab Dis 1983;6:105–106
25. Gahl WA, Renlund M, Thoene JG. Cystinosis. In: Scriver CR, Beaudet AL, Sly WS, Valle D, eds. The metabolic basis of inherited disease. New York: McGraw-Hill, 1989:2619–2635
26. Wong VG, Kuwabara T, Brubaker R, et al. Intralysosomal cystine crystal in cystinosis. Invest Ophthalmol Vis Sci 1970;9:83–88

27. Lietman PS, Frazier PD, Wong VG, et al. Adult cystinosis: a benign disorder. Am J Med 1966;40:511–517
28. Sanderson PO, Kuwabara T, Stark WJ, et al. Cystinosis. A clinical, histopathologic and ultrastructural study. Arch Ophthalmol 1974;91:270–274
29. Ketz B, Melles RB, Schneider JA. Glare disability in nephropathic cystinosis. Arch Ophthalmol 1987;105:1670–1671
30. Wong VG, Lietman PS, Seegmiller JE. Alterations of pigment epithelium in cystinosis. Arch Ophthalmol 1967;77:369
31. Dufier JL, Dhermy P, Gubler MC, et al. Ocular changes in long term evaluation of infantile cystinosis. Ophthal Paediatr Genet 1987;8:131–137
32. Gahl WA, Reed GF, Thoene JG, et al. Cysteamine therapy for children with nephropathic cystinosis. N Engl J Med 1987;316:971–977
33. Kaiser-Kupfer MI, Gazzo MA, Datiles MB, et al. A randomized placebo-controlled trial of cysteamine eyedrops in nephropathic cystinosis. Arch Ophthalmol 1990; 108:689–693
34. Wilson DP, Jelley D, Stratton R, et al. Nephropathic cystinosis: improved linear growth after treatment with recombinant human growth hormone. J Pediatr 1989;115:758–761
35. Gahl WA, Bernardini I, Dalakas M, et al. Oral carnitine therapy in children with cystinosis and Fanconi syndrome. J Clin Invest 1988;81:549–560
36. Fenton WA, Rosenberg LE. Inherited disorders of cobalamin transport and metabolism. In: Scriver CR, Beaudet AL, Sly WS, Valle D, eds. The metabolic basis of inherited disease. New York: McGraw-Hill, 1989:2065–2082
37. Brown RD, Maumenee IH. Methylmalonic aciduria and homocystinuria-A disorder of intracellular vitamin B12 metabolism. Invest Ophthalmol Vis Sci 1989; 30(suppl):307
38. Robb RM, Dowton SB, Fulton AB, et al. Retinal degeneration in vitamin B12 disorder associated with methylmalonic aciduria and sulfur amino acid abnormalities. Am J Ophthalmol 1984;97:691–696
39. Watkins D, Rosenblatt DS. Failure of lysosomal release of vitamin B12: a new complementation group causing methylmalonic aciduria (Cb1F). Am J Hum Genet 1986;39:404–408
40. Bartholomew DW, Allen RH, Roe CR, et al. Therapeutic approaches to Cbl-C methylmalonic acidemia and homocystinuria. J Pediatr 1988;1/2:32
41. Bain MD, Jones M, Borriello SP, et al. Contribution of gut bacterial metabolism to human metabolic disease. Lancet 1988;1:1078–1079
42. Bassen FA, Kornzweig AL. Malformation of the erythrocytes in a case of atypical retinitis pigmentosa. Blood 1950;5:381–387
43. Goodman RM. Genetic disorders of the Jewish people. Baltimore: Johns Hopkins University Press, 1979: 69–71
44. Salt HB, Wolff OH, Lloyd JK, et al. On having no beta-lipoprotein; a syndrome comprising abetalipoproteinemia, acanthocytosis, and steatorrhea. Lancet 1960; 2:325–329
45. Runge P, Muller DPR, McAllister J, et al. Oral vitamin E supplements can prevent the retinopathy of abetalipoproteinemia. Br J Ophthalmol 1986;70:166–173
46. Mabry CC, DiGeorge AM, Auerbach VH. Studies concerning the defect in a patient with acanthocytosis. Clin Res 1960;8:371
47. Kornzweig AL, Bassen FA. Retinitis pigmentosa, acanthocystosis, and heredodegenerative neuromuscular disease. Arch Ophthalmol 1957;58:183
48. Gouras P, Carr RE, Gunkel RD. Retinitis pigmentosa in abetalipoproteinemia: effects of vitamin A. Invest Ophthalmol 1971;10:784
49. Lamy M, Frezal J, Polonovski J, Rey J. L'absence congenitale des beta-lipoproteines. Presse Medicale 1961;69:1511
50. Muller DP, Lloyd JK, Bird AC. Long term management of abetalipoproteinemia. Possible role for vitamin E. Arch Dis Child 1977;52:209

51. Neufeld EF, Muenzer J. The mucopolysaccharidoses. In: Scriver CR, Beaudet AL, Sly WS, Valle D, eds. The metabolic basis of inherited disease. New York: McGraw-Hill, 1989:1565–1587
52. Leug L-SE, Weinstein GW, Hobson RR. Further electroretinographic studies of patients with mucopolysaccharidoses. Birth Defects 1971;7(3):32–40
53. Collins ML, Traboulsi EI, Maumenee IH. Optic nerve head swelling and optic atrophy in the mucopolysaccharidoses. Ophthalmology 1990;97:1445–1449
54. Newell FW, Koistinen A. Lipochondrodystrophy (gargoylism). Pathologic findings in five eyes of three patients. Arch Ophthalmol 1955;53:45–62
55. Chan CC, Green WR, Maumenee IH, et al. Ocular ultrastructural studies of two cases of the Hurler syndrome (systemic mucopolysaccharidosis I-H). Ophthal Paediatr Genet 1983;2:3–19
56. Del Monte M, Maumenee IH, Green WR, et al. Clinical and ocular histopathologic studies of mucopolysaccharidosis type III-A: the Sanfilippo syndrome. Arch Ophthalmol 1983;101:1255–1262
57. Lavery MA, Green WR, Jabs EW, et al. Ocular histopathology and ultrastructure of Sanfilippo's syndrome, type III-B. Arch Ophthalmol 1983;101:1263–1274
58. Amir N, Zlotogora J, Bach G. Mucolipidosis type IV; clinical spectrum and natural history. Pediatrics 1987;79:953–959
59. Reidel KG, Zwaan J, Kenyon KR, et al. Ocular abnormalities in mucolipidosis IV. Am J Ophthalmol 1985;99:125–136
60. Bach G, Zeigler M, Schaap T, et al. Mucolipidosis type IV: ganglioside sialidase deficiency. Biochem Biophys Res Commun 1979;90:1341–1347
61. Lieser M, Harms E, Kern H, et al. Ganglioside GM 3 sialidase activity in fibroblasts of normal individuals and of patients with sialisosis and mucolipidosis IV. Subcellular distribution and some properties. Biochem J 1989;260:69–74
62. Kenyon KR, Maumenee IH, Green WR, et al. Mucolipidosis IV: Histopathology of conjunctiva, cornea and skin. Arch Ophthalmol 1979;97:1106–1111
63. Dangel ME, Bremer DL, Rogers GL. Treatment of corneal opacification in mucolipidosis IV with conjunctival transplantation. Am J Ophthalmol 1985;99: 137–141
64. Poulos A, Singh H, Paton B, et al. Accumulation and defective beta-oxidation of very long chain fatty acids in Zellweger's syndrome, adrenoleukodystrophy and Refsum disease variants. Clin Genet 1986;29:397–408
65. Wilson GN, Holmes PD, Hajra AK. Peroxisomal disorders: clinical commentary and future prospects. Am J Med Genet 1988;30:771–792
66. Lambert SR, Kriss A, Taylor D, et al. Follow-up and diagnostic reappraisal of 75 patients with Leber's congenital amaurosis. Am J Ophthalmol 1989;107:624–631
67. Moser HW. Peroxisomal disorders. J Pediatr 1986;108:89–91
68. Bowen P, Lee CSN, Zellweger H, et al. A familial syndrome of multiple congenital defects. Bull Johns Hopkins Hosp 1964;114:402
69. Garner A, Fielder AR, Primavesi R, et al. Tapetoretinal degeneration in the cerebro-hepato-renal (Zellweger's) syndrome. Br J Ophthalmol 1982;66:422
70. Cohen SMZ, Brown FR III, Martyn L, et al. Ocular histopathologic and biochemical studies of the cerebrohepatorenal (Zellweger's) syndrome and its relationship to neonatal adrenoleukodystrophy. Am J Ophthalmol 1983;96:488–501
71. Kelley RI, Datta NS, Dobyns WB, et al. Neonatal adrenoleukodystrophy: new cases, biochemical studies, and differentiation from Zellweger and related peroxisomal polydystrophy syndrome. Am J Med Genet 1986;23:869–901
72. Cohen SMZ, Green WR, delaCruz ZC, et al. Ocular histopathologic studies of neonatal and childhood adrenoleukodystrophy. Am J Ophthalmol 1983;95: 82–96
73. Glasgow BJ, Brown HH, Hannah JB, et al. Ocular pathologic findings in neonatal adrenoleukodystrophy. Ophthalmology 1987;94:1054–1060
74. Refsum S. Heredopathia atactica polyneuritiformis. Phytanic acid storage dis-

ease, Refsum's disease: a biochemically well-defined disease with a specific dietary treatment. Arch Neurol 1981;38:605–606
75. Hansen E, Bachen NI, Flage T. Refsum's disease: eye manifestations in a patient treated with low phytol low phytanic acid diet. Acta Ophthalmol (Copenh) 1979; 57:382–396
76. Scotto JM, Hadchouel M, Odievre M, et al. Infantile phytamic acid storage disease, a possible variant of Refsum's disease. Three cases, including ultrastructural studies of the liver. J Inherit Dis 1982;5:83–90
77. Weleber RG, Tongue AC, Kennaway NG, et al. Ophthalmic manifestations of infantile phytanic acid storage disease. Arch Ophthalmol 1984;102:1307–1321
78. Zeman W. Studies in the neuronal ceroid lipofuscinoses. Presidential address. J Neuropathol Exp Neurol 1974;33:1–12
79. Boustany R-MN, Kolodny EH. The neuronal ceroid lipofuscinoses: a review. Rev Neurol (Paris) 1989;142:105–110
80. Traboulsi EI, Green WR, de la Cruz ZC, et al. The neuronal ceroid lipofuscinoses. Ocular histopathologic studies in the late infantile, juvenile and adult forms. Graefes Arch Clin Exp Ophthalmol 1987;225:391–402
81. Bateman BR, Philippart M. Ocular features of the Hagberg-Santavuori syndrome. Am J Ophthalmol 1986;102:262–271
82. Hagberg B, Witt-Engerstrom I. Early stages of Rett syndrome and infantile neuronal ceroid lipofuscinosis—a difficult differential diagnosis. Brain Dev 1990; 12:20–22
83. Jarvela I, Maenpaa J, Haataja L, et al. Assignment of infantile form of neuronal ceroid lipofuscinosis (INCL) to the short arm of chromosome 1. Am J Hum Genet 1990;47(suppl):185
84. Raitta C, Santavuori P. Ophthalmological findings in the infantile type of so-called neuronal ceroid-lipofuscinosis. Acta Ophthalmol (Copenh) 1973;51:755–763
85. Dom R, Brucher JM, Ceuterick C, et al. Adult ceroid lipofuscinosis (Kufs' disease) in two brothers. Retinal and visceral storage in one; diagnostic muscle biopsy in the other. Acta Neuropathol (Berl) 1979;45:67–72
86. Brod RD, Packer AJ, Van Dyk HJL. Diagnosis of neuronal ceroid lipofuscinosis by ultrastructural examination of peripheral blood lymphocytes. Arch Ophthalmol 1987;105:1388–1393
87. MacLeod PM, Dolman CL, Nickel RE, et al. Prenatal diagnosis of neuronal ceroid lipofuscinosis. N Engl J Med 1984;310:595
88. Rapola J, Santavuori P, Heiska H. Placental pathology and prenatal diagnosis of infantile type of NCL. Am J Hum Genet 1988;5:99–103
89. Harding AE. Classification of the hereditary ataxias and paraplegias. Lancet 1983;1:1151–1154
90. Koenigsmark BW, Weiner LP. The olivopontocerebellar atrophies: a review. Medicine 1970;49:227–241
91. Amit R, Granit G, Shapira Y. Familial ataxia with extreme difference in age of clinical onset. Neuropediatrics 1986;17:165–167
92. Traboulsi EI, Maumenee IH, Green WR, et al. Olivopontocerebellar atrophy with retinal degeneration. A clinical and ocular histopathologic study. Arch Ophthalmol 1988;106:801–806
93. Ryan SJ, Smith RE. Retinopathy associated with hereditary olivopontocerebellar degeneration. Am J Ophthalmol 1971;71:838–843
94. de Jong PTVM, de Jong JGY, de Jong-Ten Doeschate JMM, et al. Olivopontocerebellar atrophy with visual disturbances. An ophthalmologic investigation into four generations. Ophthalmology 1980;87:793–804
95. Ryan SJ, Knox DL, Green WR, Konigsmark BW. Olivopontocerebellar degeneration. Clinicopathologic correlation of the associated retinopathy. Arch Ophthalmol 1975;93:169–172

96. Kearns TP, Sayre GP. Retinitis pigmentosa, external ophthalmoplegia, and complete heart block. Arch Ophthalmol 1958;60:280–289
97. Bastiaensen LAK. Pigment changes of the retina in chronic progressive external ophthalmoplegia. Acta Ophthalmol (Copenh) 1978;56(suppl 138):5–36
98. Eagle RC Jr, Hedges TR, Yanoff M. The atypical pigmentary retinopathy of Kearns-Sayre syndrome. Ophthalmology 1982;89:1433–1440
99. Bosche J, Hammerstein W, Neuen-Jacob E, Schober R. Variation in retinal changes and muscle pathology in mitochondriopathies. Graefes Arch Clin Exp Ophthalmol 1989;227:578–583
100. Moraes CT, DiMauro S, Zeviani M, et al. Mitochondrial DNA deletions in progressive external ophthalmoplegia and Kearns-Sayre syndrome. N Engl J Med 1989; 320:1293–1299
101. Rowland LP, Hausmanowa-Petrusewicz I, Bardurska B, et al. Kearns-Sayre syndrome in twins: lethal dominant mutation or acquired disease? Neurology (NY) 1988;38:1399–1402
102. Schnitzler ER, Robertson EC Jr. Familial Kearns-Sayre syndrome. Neurology (NY) 1979;29:1172–1174
103. Leveille AS, Newell FW. Autosomal dominant Kearns-Sayre syndrome. Ophthalmology 1980;87:99–108
104. Pericak-Vance MA, Yamaoka LH, Assinder RIF, et al. Tight linkage of apolipoprotein C2 to myotonic dystrophy on chromosome 19. Neurology (NY) 1986; 36:1418–1423
105. Betten MG, Bilchik RC, Smith ME. Pigmentary retinopathy of myotonic dystrophy. Am J Ophthalmol 1971;72:720–723
106. Stanescu B, Michiels J. Temporal aspects of electroretinography in patients with myotonic dystrophy. Am J Ophthalmol 1975;80:224–226
107. Raitta C, Karli P. Ocular findings in myotonic dystrophy. Ann Ophthalmol 1982;14:647–650
108. Walker SD, Brubaker RF, Nagatoki S. Hypotony and aqueous humor dynamics in myotonic dystrophy. Invest Ophthalmol Vis Sci 1982;22:744–751
109. Dooling EC, Schoene WC, Richardson EP Jr. Hallervorden-Spatz syndrome. Arch Neurol 1974;30:70
110. Murphy MA, Feldman JA, Kilburn G. Hallervorden-Spatz in a psychiatric setting. J Clin Psychiatry 1989;50:66–68
111. Schaffert DA, Johnsen SD, Johnson PC, et al. Magnetic resonance imaging in pathologically proven Hallervorden-Spatz disease. Neurology (NY) 1989;39: 440–442
112. Galluci M, Cardona F, Arachi M, et al. Follow-up MR studies in Hallervorden-Spatz disease. J Comput Assist Tomogr 1990;14:118–120
113. Luckenback MW, Green WR, Miller NR, et al. Ocular clinicopathologic correlation of Hallervorden-Spatz syndrome with acanthocytosis and pigmentary retinopathy. Am J Ophthalmol 1983;95:369–382
114. Eidelberg D, Sotrel A, Joachim C, et al. Adult-onset Hallervorden-Spatz disease with neurofibrillary pathology. A discrete clinicopathological entity. Brain 1987; 110:993–1013
115. Newell RW, Johnson RO II, Huttenlocher PR. Pigmentary degeneration of the retina in the Hallervorden-Spatz syndrome. Am J Ophthalmol 1979;88:467–471
116. Roth AM, Helper RS, Mukoyama M, et al. Pigmentary retinal dystrophy in Hallervorden-Spatz disease: clinicopathological report of a case. Surv Ophthalmol 1971;16:24–35
117. Joubert M, Eisenring J, Andermann F. Familial agenesis of the cerebellar vermis. Neurology (NY) 1969;19:813–825
118. Lambert SR, Kriss A, Gresty M, et al. Joubert syndrome. Arch Ophthalmol 1989;107:709–713

119. Flynn A, Aird RB. A neuroectodermal syndrome of dominant inheritance. J Neurol Sci 1965;2:161–182
120. Itin P, Buchner SA, Gloor B. Darier's disease and retinitis pigmentosa; is there a pathogenetic relationship? Br J Dermatol 1988;119:397–402
121. Elliott S, Buxman M, Weleber R. Abnormal dark adaptation in Darier's disease. J Invest Dermatol 1979;72:207
122. Senior B. Familial renal-retinal dystrophy. Am J Dis Child 1973;125:442–447
123. Betts P, Forrest-Hay I. Juvenile nephronophthisis. Lancet 1978;2:475–478
124. Senior B, Friedman A, Brando J. Juvenile familial nephropathy with tapetoretinal degeneration. Am J Ophthalmol 1961;52:625–633
125. Fairley K, Leighton P. Familial visual defects associated with polycystic kidney and medullary sponge kidney. Br Med J 1963;1:1060–1063
126. Hussels I. Congenital amaurosis and nephronophthisis: a new syndrome. Birth Defects 1971;7(3):199
127. Polak B, Hogewind B, Van Lith F. Tapetoretinal degeneration associated with recessively inherited medullary cystic disease. Am J Ophthalmol 1977;84:645–651
128. Dekaban A. Hereditary syndrome of congenital retinal blindness (Leber), polycystic kidneys and maldevelopment of the brain. Am J Ophthalmol 1969;68: 1029–1037
129. Fernandez-Rodriguez R, Morales JM, Martinez R, et al. Senior-Loken syndrome (nephronophthisis and pigmentary retinopathy) associated with liver fibrosis: a family study. Nephron 1990;55:74–77
130. Godel V, Iaina A, Nemet P, Lazar M. Retinal manifestations in familial juvenile nephronophthisis. Clin Genet 1979;16:277–281
131. Bard LA, Bard PA, Owens GW, Hall BD. Retinal involvement in thoracic pelvic phalangeal dystrophy. Arch Ophthalmol 1978;96:278
132. Wilson DJ, Weleber RG, Beals RK. Retinal dystrophy in Jeune's syndrome. Arch Ophthalmol 1987;105:651–657
133. Allen AW, Moon JB, Hovland KR, Mickler DS. Ocular findings in thoracic-pelvic-phalangeal dystrophy. Arch Ophthalmol 1979;97:489
134. Cockayne EA. Dwarfism with retinal atrophy and deafness. Arch Dis Child 1946;21:52–54
135. Otsuka F, Robbins JH. The Cockayne syndrome—an inherited multisystem disorder with cutaneous photosensitivity and defective repair of DNA. Am J Dermatopathol 1985;7:387–392
136. Coles W. Ocular manifestations of Cockayne's syndrome. Am J Ophthalmol 1969;67:762–764
137. Pearce WG. Ocular and genetic features of Cockayne's syndrome. Can J Ophthalmol 1972;7:435–444
138. Brodrick JD, Dark AJ. Corneal dystrophy in Cockayne's syndrome. Br J Ophthalmol 1973;57:391–399
139. Green JS, Parfrey PS, Harnett JD, et al. The cardinal manifestations of Bardet-Biedl syndrome. N Engl J Med 1989;321:1002–1009
140. Churchill DN, McManamon P, Hurley RM. Renal disease: a sixth cardinal feature of the Laurence-Moon-Biedl syndrome. Clin Nephrol 1981;16:151–154
141. Harnett JD, Green JS, Cramer BC, et al. The spectrum of renal disease in Laurence-Moon-Biedl syndrome. N Engl J Med 1988;319:615–618
142. Escallon F, Traboulsi EI, Infante R. A family with the Bardet-Biedl syndrome and diabetes mellitus. Arch Ophthalmol 1989;107:855–857
143. Farag TI, Teebi AS. High incidence of Bardet-Biedl syndrome among the Bedouin. Clin Genet 1989;36:463–465
144. Schachat AP, Maumenee IH. Bardet-Biedl syndrome and related disorders. Arch Ophthalmol 1982;100:285–288

145. Leys MJ, Schreiner LA, Hansen RM, et al. Visual acuities and dark-adapted thresholds of children with Bardet-Biedl syndrome. Am J Ophthalmol 1988; 106:561–569
146. Jacobson SG, Borruat F-X, Apathy PP. Patterns of rod and cone dysfunction in Bardet-Biedl syndrome. Am J Ophthalmol 1990;109:676–688
147. Ruben JB, Morris RJ, Judisch GF. Chorioretinal degeneration in infantile malignant osteopetrosis. Am J Ophthalmol 1990;110:1–5
148. Fishman GA, Kumar A, Joseph ME, et al. Usher's syndrome. Ophthalmic and neuro-otologic findings suggesting genetic heterogeneity. Arch Ophthalmol 1983;101:1367–1374
149. Hallgren B. Retinitis pigmentosa combined with congenital deafness; with vestibulo-cerebellar ataxia and mental abnormality in a proportion of cases. A clinical and genetico-statistical study. Acta Psychiatr Scand [Suppl] 1959;138: 5–101
150. Lewis RA, Otterud B, Stauffer D, et al. Mapping recessive ophthalmic diseases: linkage of the locus for Usher syndrome type II to a DNA marker on chromosome 1q. Genomics 1990;7:250–256
151. Piazza L, Fishman GA, Farmer M, et al. Visual acuity loss in patients with Usher's syndrome. Arch Ophthalmol 1986;104:1336–1339
152. Bloom TD, Fishman GA, Mafee MF. Usher's syndrome. CNS defects determined by computed tomography. Retina 1983;3:108–113
153. Hunter DG, Fishman GA, Mehta RS, et al. Abnormal sperm and photoreceptor axonemes in Usher's syndrome. Am J Ophthalmol 1986;104:385–399
154. Bateman JB, Riedner ED, Levin LS, et al. Heterogeneity of retinal degeneration and hearing impairment syndromes. Am J Ophthalmol 1980;90:755–767
155. Alstrom CH, Hallgren B, Nilsson LB, Asander H. Retinal degeneration combined with obesity, diabetes mellitus and neurogenous deafness: a specific syndrome (not hitherto described) distinct from the Laurence-Moon-Bardet-Biedl syndrome. Acta Psychiatr Neurol Scand [Suppl] 1959;129:1–35
156. Millay RH, Weleber RG, Heckenlively JR. Ophthalmologic and systemic manifestations of Alstrom's disease. Am J Ophthalmol 1986;102:482–490
157. Sebag J, Albert DM, Craft JL. The Alstrom syndrome: ophthalmic histopathology and retinal ultrastructure. Br J Ophthalmol 1984;68:494–501
158. Mueller RF: The Alagille syndrome (arteriohepatic dysplasia). J Med Genet 1987;24:621–626
159. Byrne JLB, Harrod MJE, Friedman JM, et al. Del (20p) with manifestations of arteriohepatic dysplasia. Am J Med Genet 1986;24:673–678
160. Puklin JE, Riely CA, Simon RM, Cotlier E. Anterior segment and retinal pigmentary abnormalities in arteriohepatic dysplasia. Ophthalmology 1981;88:337–347
161. Traboulsi EI, Lustbader J, Lemp MA. Keratoconus in Alagille syndrome. Am J Ophthalmol 1989;108:332–333
162. Johnson BL. Ocular pathologic features of arteriohepatic dysplasia (Alagille's syndrome). Am J Ophthalmol 1990;110:504–512
163. O'Neill JF, Drack AV. Rubella—German measles. In: Gold DH, Weingeist TA, eds. The eye in systemic disease. Philadelphia: Lippincott, 1990:269–272
164. Pulido JS, Corbett JJ, McLeish WM. Syphilis. In: Gold DH, Weingeist TA, eds. The eye in systemic disease. Philadelphia: Lippincott, 1990:233–239

Systemic Associations of Angioid Streaks

Ahmad M. Mansour, M.D.

Angioid streaks have a characteristic appearance of linear, narrow subretinal streaks radiating a few millimeters from a peripapillary ring (Fig 1). Angioid streaks appear in the second decade of life and are usually bilateral. The length, width, and number of the streaks is variable. The color of the streaks varies from red and gray (so-called fresh streaks) to yellow (atrophic streaks) [1]. There is a high incidence of macular degeneration at a young age in eyes with angioid streaks (Fig 2). Macular subretinal neovascular membrane formation and visual loss occur in more than 50% of eyes with angioid streaks [1]. Subretinal neovascular membranes (Fig 3) usually arise at the edge of one of the angioid streaks and, less commonly, outside the streak in the macular region or in a peripapillary location (especially with the presence of optic disc drusen). More than one-third of eyes with angioid streaks display a prominent mottled fundus (also called *peau d'orange,* or orange-peel, appearance). Approximately 10% of eyes with angioid streaks have the diffuse type, or the cracked eggshell appearance. In this diffuse variety, the streaks are not only radial but are also concentric, forming a mosaic of streaks. The diffuse variety carries a poor visual prognosis because of commonly occurring disciform scarring of the macula. Eyes with angioid streaks are susceptible to subretinal hemorrhaging on minor ocular trauma, usually around the streaks [1]. By fluorescein angiography, the streaks either display early hyperfluorescence (fresh streaks) or early hypofluorescence (atrophic streaks) [1], with uniformly late hyperfluorescence (Fig 4). The streaks may widen and lengthen. The end stage includes disciform macular degeneration, helicoid peripapillary atrophy (around the streaks), and diffuse chorioretinal degeneration (with effacement of the streaks).

Histopathologically, angioid streaks correspond to a full-thickness break in Bruch's membrane with disruption of the underlying choriocapillaris and atrophy of the overlying retinal pigment epithelium [2] (Fig 5). Bruch's membrane is also thickened and basophilic and contains calcium. Secondary atrophy of the choriocapillaris and of the overlying retinal pigment epithelium occurs at the area of the streak.

Nearly half of subjects with angioid streaks have an associated underlying systemic disorder, whereas remaining subjects have idiopathic angioid streaks

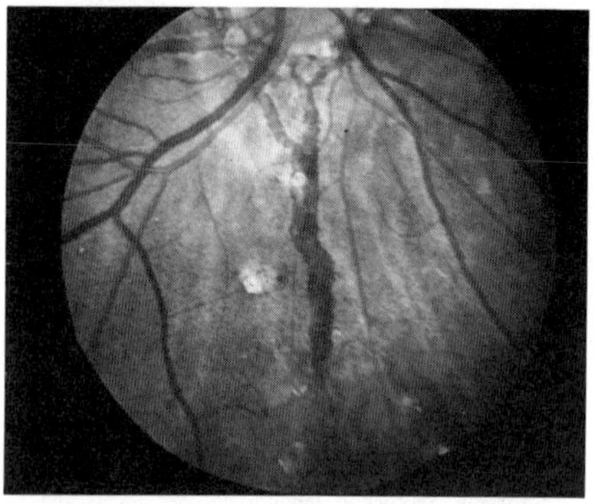

Figure 1 *Radial linear streaks emanating from the disc margins are characteristic of angioid streaks. Large drusen of the retinal pigment epithelium are noted and are surrounded by a comet-shaped area of hypopigmented retinal pigment epithelium.*

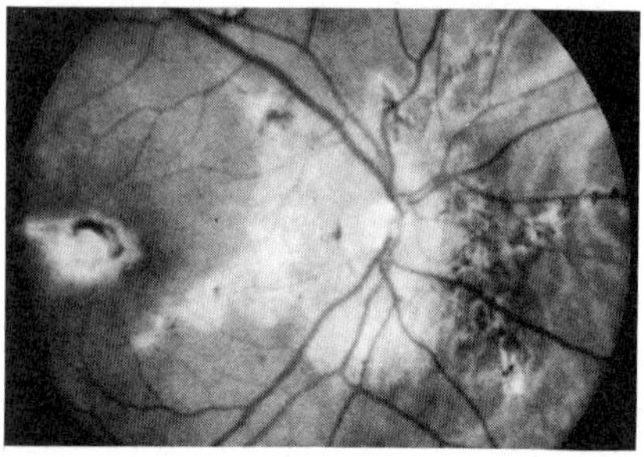

Figure 2 *Disciform macular degeneration in an eye with angioid streaks.*

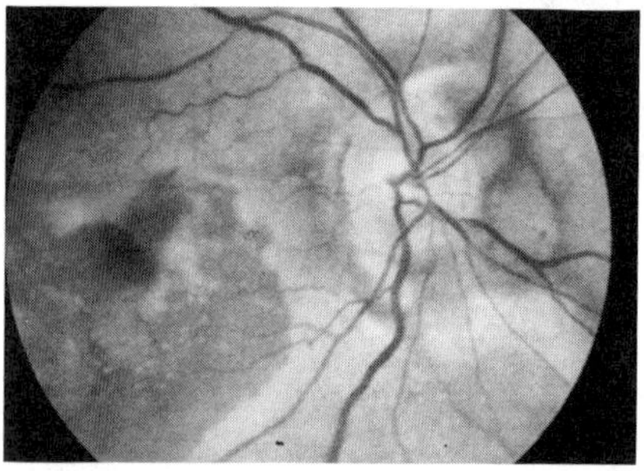

Figure 3 *Subretinal hemorrhage from a subretinal neovascular membrane in the macular region. Angioid streaks are noted around disc.*

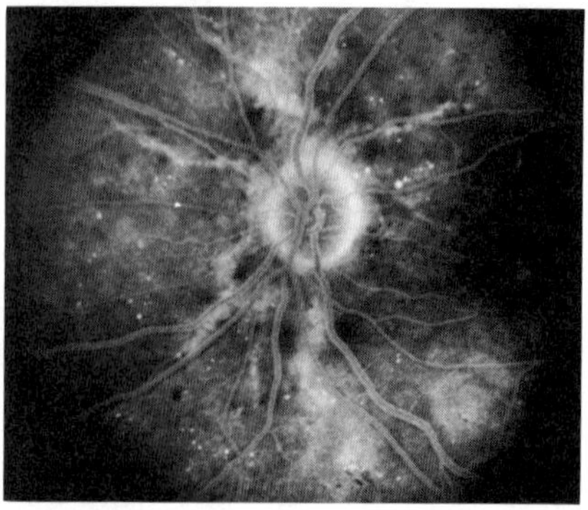

Figure 4 *Fine linear streaks showing late hyperfluorescence in a patient with background diabetic retinopathy.*

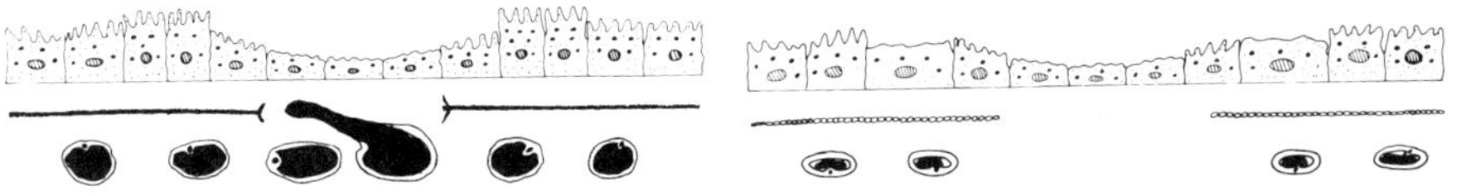

A B

Figure 5 *Pathological changes in angioid streaks: break in Bruch's membrane, overlying atrophy of the retinal pigment epithelium, and underlying subretinal neovascular membrane (A) or atrophy of the underlying choriocapillaris (B).*

[3, 4]. Established systemic associations with angioid streaks are described (Table 1), excluding coincidental occurrences (i.e., neurofibromatosis, diffuse lipomatosis, familial polyposis, lead poisoning, Sturge-Weber syndrome, tuberous sclerosis, and systemic lupus erythematosus) [3, 5]. Three major categories (dermatological, hematological, and osteogenic) of systemic disorders are associated with angioid streaks.

■ Pseudoxanthoma Elasticum

The most common disorder associated with angioid streaks is pseudoxanthoma elasticum, an inherited disorder of connective tissue. It is an underdiagnosed, genetically heterogeneous disorder with protean manifestations. The disorder derives its name from the characteristic xanthomalike papular and reticulated skin lesions (plucked-chicken appearance in neck and axillae) (Fig 6) [6]. Other manifestations include occlusive peripheral and coronary artery disease, upper gastrointestinal tract hemorrhage, and hypertension [6,

Table 1 *Systemic Disorders Associated with Angioid Streaks*

System Affected	Disorder	Order of Frequency*
Skin	Pseudoxanthoma elasticum (Grönblad-Strandberg syndrome)	1
	Fibrodysplasia Hyperelastica (Ehlers-Danlos syndrome)	6
	Senile elastosis	4
Bone	Paget's disease of bone (osteitis deformans)	2
	Chronic congenital idiopathic hyperphosphatasemia (juvenile Paget's disease of bone)	8
	Calcinosis	10
	Acromegaly	11
Blood	Sickle cell hemoglobinopathies	3
	Thalassemia	5
	Acanthocytosis (abetalipoproteinemia; Bassen-Kornzweig syndrome)	7
	Hereditary spherocytosis	9

*1 = most frequent, 11 = least frequent.

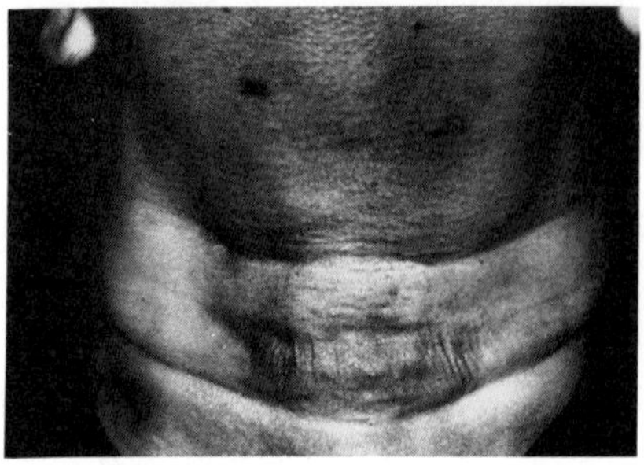

Figure 6 *Plucked-chicken appearance of skin of the neck in a middle-aged black woman. Angioid streaks were discovered on routine examination, and the diagnosis of pseudoxanthoma elasticum was subsequently made.*

7] (Fig 7). The basic pathogenetic lesion is believed to be a defect in the elastic fibers from abnormal collagen or abnormal elastin [8]. The prevalence of pseudoxanthoma elasticum is approximately 1:160,000. More than 50% of subjects with angioid streaks have pseudoxanthoma elasticum [4], and this percentage is expected to be higher if cases of subclinical pseudoxanthoma elasticum are diagnosed and counted [9]. Angioid streaks are detected in more than 90% of subjects with pseudoxanthoma elasticum [10]. Subclinical cases of pseudoxanthoma elasticum are diagnosed by skin biopsy, with findings of swollen, fragmented, irregularly clumped elastic fibers in the middermis (Fig 8). The severity of elastic fiber degeneration histologically correlates with the clinical appearance of the skin but does not correlate with the presence of angioid streaks [9].

■ Paget's Disease

The second most common disorder is Paget's disease of bone. In this disease, gross deformities of the skull, pelvis, and spine are associated with pain, elevation of serum alkaline phosphatase, and elevated urine total peptide hydroxyproline [3]. The disorder is characterized by development of coarsely trabeculated, calcified, and thickened sclerotic bone (evident radiographically)

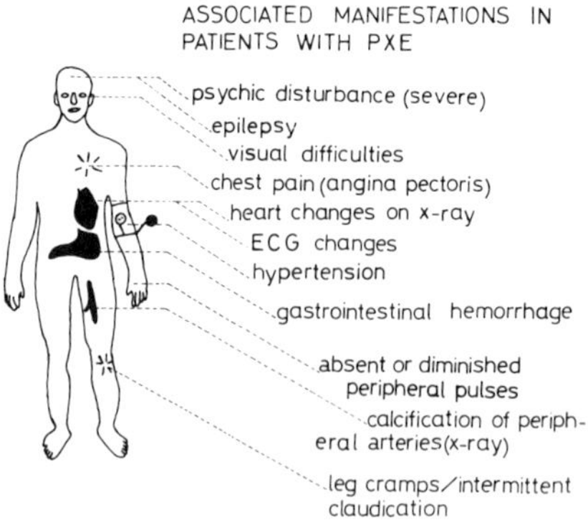

Figure 7 *Systemic manifestations in pseudoxanthoma elasticum. (ECG = electrocardiogram.)*

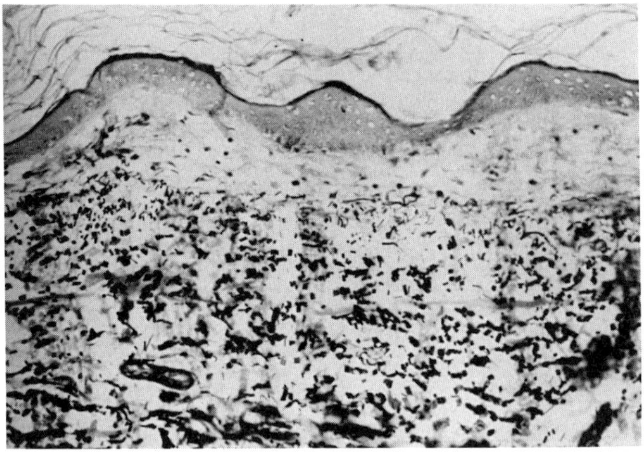

Figure 8 *Skin biopsy in a patient with pseudoxanthoma elasticum demonstrates fragmented, curly, darkly staining elastic fibers in the mid-dermis (elastic von Gieson stain).*

from uncontrolled primary osteoclastic response. Similarities with pseudoxanthoma elasticum include presence of angioid streaks [11] and calcification of medium-sized arteries. Paget's osteitis deformans is present with variable degrees of severity in up to 4% of the elderly population [12]. Approximately 2% of subjects with angioid streaks have Paget's disease of bone [1], whereas 14% of subjects with active and manifest Paget's disease of bone have angioid streaks [3].

■ Other Systemic Diseases

Patients with sickle cell hemoglobinopathies account for 1% of subjects with angioid streaks. Angioid streaks have been described in sickle cell disease, sickle cell trait, sickle cell thalassemia, sickle cell hemoglobin C disease, alpha-thalassemia, and beta-thalassemia [3, 13–16]. Elastic tissue degeneration was documented in sickle cell hemoglobinopathies [15].

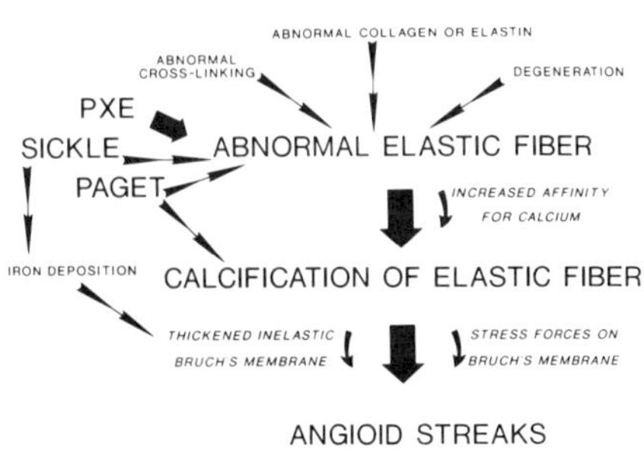

Figure 9 *Proposed pathogenetic mechanisms of angioid streak formation in various systemic disorders. (PXE = pseudoxanthoma elasticum; SICKLE = sickle cell hemoglobinopathies; PAGET = Paget's disease.)*

Table 2 *Major Systemic Diseases Affecting the Elastic Fiber*

Pseudoxanthoma elasticum
Elastosis perforans serpiginosa
Cutis laxa
Menkes' kinky-hair syndrome
Ehlers-Danlos syndrome (type V)
Marfan's syndrome
Copper deficiency
Senile elastosis

Less frequent systemic disorders associated with angioid streaks include abetalipoproteinemia [17], hereditary spherocytosis [18], Ehlers-Danlos syndrome [19], calcinosis [20], juvenile Paget's disease of bone (chronic familial hyperphosphatasemia) [21], and senile elastosis.

■ Possible Pathogenetic Link Between Angioid Streaks and Systemic Disease

My colleagues and I propose the following pathogenetic link between angioid streaks and the various associated systemic disorders (Fig 9). In the systemic disorders listed in Table 2, the elastic tissues express variable degrees of abnormality [15]. This abnormality increases the affinity toward calcium, leading to calcification of elastic fibers [8]. Histopathologically, Bruch's membrane has an elastic core and two collagenous layers on each side of the central elastic layer [22]. The elastic tissue of Bruch's membrane is connected to the choroidal elastic tissue and to the ciliary epithelium [23]. In pseudoxanthoma elasticum, Bruch's membrane is thickened and calcified [24], as it is in eyes with angioid streaks and Paget's disease [11] or with angioid streaks and sickle cell hemoglobinopathies [13, 14]. The brittleness of Bruch's membrane in sickle disorders is attributed to calcification [25] rather than to iron deposition [14], which was not present uniformly in such eyes [25]. Inelastic, calcified, and thickened Bruch's membrane is submitted to the mechanical stretching of the extraocular muscles (with the base of the vector forces being at the peripapillary ring) [26, 27], leading to radial breaks in Bruch's membrane. The angioid streaks are limited to the posterior pole and start around the disc margin. In blunt ocular trauma in experimental animals, the transmission of energy forces occur along the walls of the globe [28], and any point where discontinuity in the wall exists or an attachment is present will be most susceptible for stress [29]. The attachment of the optic nerve head and of the posterior ciliaries make the posterior pole vulnerable to increased stress and stretch forces. The factors leading to rupture of Bruch's membrane are not well elucidated but may include repetitive minor ocular trauma (such as forceful rubbing of the eyes) and acute blunt ocular trauma. Breaks in Bruch's membrane occur in age-related macular degeneration (rupture of the retinal pigment epithelium is more common than rupture of Bruch's membrane, such as in age-related retinal pigment epithelial detachments [30]), choroiditis (macrophages destroying the membrane, such as in presumed ocular histoplasmosis syndrome, or ocular toxoplasmosis), choroidal rupture (concentric forces involving primarily the choroid [29]), and high myopia [27]. In high myopia, Bruch's membrane is thinned out and gapes in areas of excessive staphylomatous formation, leading to a few small linear lacquer cracks. The mechanism of rupture of Bruch's membrane in angioid streaks (thickening of Bruch's membrane, which cracks by stress forces) is quite the opposite of that in high myopia (effacement of Bruch's membrane that gapes secondary to ectasia of surrounding tissue).

■ Diagnostic Workup

Workup of subjects with angioid streaks who lack the signs and symptoms of established systemic disorders include radiography of skull, abdomen, and lower extremities, determination of serum alkaline phosphatase, calcium, and phosphorus levels, hemoglobin electrophoresis, and skin biopsy [3]. Angioid streaks represent a local sign of a generalized disorder of connective tissue, namely of the elastic fiber, and present predominantly in the context of pseudoxanthoma elasticum, Paget's disease of bone, and sickle cell hemoglobinopathies.

■ References

1. Mansour AM, Shields JA, Annesley WH, et al. Macular degeneration in angioid streaks. Ophthalmologica 1988;197:36
2. Dreyer R, Green WR. The pathology of angioid streaks: a study of twenty-one cases. Trans Pa Acad Ophthalmol Otolaryngol 1978;31:158
3. Clarkson JG, Altman RD. Angioid streaks. Surv Ophthalmol 1982;26:235
4. Shields JA, Federman JL, Tomer TL, et al. Angioid streaks: I. Ophthalmoloscopic variations and diagnostic problems. Br J Ophthalmol 1975;59:257
5. Awan KJ. Familial polyposis and angioid streaks in the ocular fundus. Am J Ophthalmol 1977;83:123
6. Eddy DD, Farber EM. Pseudoxanthoma elasticum; internal manifestations, a report of cases and a statistical review of the literature. Arch Dermatol 1962;86:729
7. Goodman RM, Smith EW, Paton D, et al. Pseudoxanthoma elasticum: a clinical and histopathological study. Medicine (Baltimore) 1963;42:297
8. McKusick V. Pseudoxanthoma elasticum. In: Heritable disorders of connective tissue. St Louis: Mosby, 1972:475–520
9. Altman LK, Fialkow PJ, Parker F, et al. Pseudoxanthoma elasticum; an underdiagnosed genetically heterogeneous disorder with protean manifestations. Arch Intern Med 1974;134:1048
10. Carlborg V, Ejrup B, Gronblad E, et al. Vascular studies in pseudoxanthoma elasticum and angioid streaks with a series of color photographs of the eyeground lesions. Acta Med Scand [Suppl] 1959;350:1
11. Gass JDM, Clarkson JG. Angioid streaks and disciform macular detachment in Paget's disease (osteitis deformans). Am J Ophthalmol 1973;75:576
12. Reasbeck JC, Goulding A, Campbell DR, et al. Radiological prevalence of Paget's disease in Dunedin, New Zealand. Br Med J 1983;286:1937

13. Geeraets WJ, Guerry DP III. Angioid streaks and sickle cell disease. Am J Ophthalmol 1960;49:450
14. Paton D. Angioid streaks and sickle cell anemia. Arch Ophthalmol 1959;62:852
15. Geeraets WJ, Guerry DP III. Elastic tissue degeneration in sickle cell disease. Am J Ophthalmol 1960;50:213
16. Gartaganis S, Ismiridis K, Papageorgiou O, et al. Ocular abnormalities in patients with beta thalassemia. Am J Ophthalmol 1989;108:699
17. Dieckert JP, White M, Christmann L, et al. Angioid streaks associated with abetalipoproteinemia. Am J Ophthalmol 1989;21:173
18. McLane NJ, Grizzard WS, Kousseff BG, et al. Angioid streaks associated with hereditary spherocytosis. Am J Ophthalmol 1984;97:444
19. Green WR, Friedman-Kien A, Banfield WG. Angioid streaks in Ehlers-Danlos syndrome. Arch Ophthalmol 1966;76:197
20. McPhaul JJ Jr, Engel FL. Heterotopic calcification, hyperphosphatemia and angioid streaks of the retina. Am J Med 1961;31:488
21. Iancu TC, Almagor G, Savir H. Ocular abnormalities in chronic familial hyperphosphatasemia. J Pediatr Ophthalmol Strabismus 1980;17:220
22. Das A, Frank RN, Zhang NL, et al. Ultrastructural localization of extracellular matrix components in human retinal vessels and Bruch's membrane. Arch Ophthalmol 1990;108:421
23. Korte GE, D'Aversa G. The elastic tissue of Bruch's membrane: connections to choroidal elastic tissue and the ciliary epithelium of the rabbit and human eyes. Arch Ophthalmol 1989;107:1654
24. Jensen OA. Bruch's membrane in pseudoxanthoma elasticum. Albrecht von Graefes Arch Klin Exp Ophthalmol 1977;203:157
25. Jampol LM, Acheson R, Eagle RC, et al. Calcification of Bruch's membrane in angioid streaks with homozygous sickle cell disease. Arch Ophthalmol 1987;105:93
26. Brazitikos PD, Safran AB. Helicoid peripapillary chorioretinal degeneration. Am J Ophthalmol 1990;109:209
27. Klein RM, Green S. The development of lacquer cracks in pathologic myopia. Am J Ophthalmol 1988;106:282
28. Delori F, Pomerantzeff O, Cox MS. Deformation of the globe under high speed impact: its relation to contusion injuries. Invest Ophthalmol 1969;8:290
29. Wood CM, Richardson J. Indirect choroidal ruptures: aetiological factors, patterns of ocular damage, and final visual outcome. Br J Ophthalmol 1990;74:208
30. Krishan NR, Chandra SR, Stevens TS. Diagnosis and pathogenesis of retinal pigment epithelial tears. Am J Ophthalmol 1985;100:698

Systemic Associations of Dry-Eye Syndrome

Ian Kaden, M.D.
Martin Mayers, M.D.

Dry-eye syndrome is a feature of many systemic illnesses and therapies. In some instances, finding dry eyes will lead the ophthalmologist, internist, or other medical care provider to suspect and further investigate a systemic disease. Sjögren and Bloch [1] estimated that 60% of the patients they followed with the sicca complex had an associated connective tissue disease. Familiarity with the spectrum of systemic illness associated with dry-eye syndrome may lead to the detection of a systemic illness early in its course.

■ Clinical Features of Dry-Eye Syndrome

Dry-eye syndrome is a common diagnosis in ophthalmic practice. A healthy tear film requires the proper balance of mucin, aqueous, and lipid components. Mucin, produced by goblet cells, provides a hydrophilic coat over the otherwise hydrophobic corneal epithelial surface. The lipid layer, elaborated by the meibomian glands and the glands of Zeis and Moll, interfaces with the atmosphere and reduces evaporation from the sandwiched aqueous layer. The middle aqueous layer comprises the bulk of the tear film and is produced by the lacrimal gland and by the accessory glands of Krause and Wolfring. Although aqueous tear deficiency (keratoconjunctivitis sicca [KCS]) is most common, a deficiency of any component of the precorneal tear film will destabilize it and can produce dry-eye syndrome.

Characteristically, patients with dry eyes complain, to varying degrees, of ocular discomfort, blurred vision, redness, and discharge. Particular levels of ocular discomfort may range from a mild awareness of one's eyes and desire to rub (itch), to a sandy or gritty foreign-body sensation, to burning, photophobia, or frank pain. These symptoms may be aggravated by smoke, chemical vapors, and cold drafts. Exposure to dry indoor heating may result in wintertime exacerbations. The blurred vision is more pronounced when a reduced blink rate allows the cornea to desiccate further. Reading or staring at a computer monitor or television screen tends to reduce the blink rate. Discharge varies from watery to mucoid. What appears to the patient as a paradoxical excessive reflex tearing occurs in less severe stages of dry-eye syndrome. Finally, when even the reflex tear secretion has become inadequate, goblet cell hypersecretion results in thick mucous strands.

Findings on slit-lamp examination can include papillary conjunctivitis; scant tear meniscus filled with cellular and mucous debris; rapid tear breakup time [BUT]; punctate epitheliopathy involving interpalpebral conjunctiva and cornea; superior limbic keratoconjunctivitis; and filamentary keratopathy. Rose bengal 1% solution is a most useful clinical stain for highlighting the range and degree of the epitheliopathy. Interpalpebral rose bengal staining can be graded as per van Bijsterveld [2]. Topical anesthetics and previous manipulation (e.g., tonometry or Schirmer strip testing) will result in artifactual rose bengal staining. Similarly, tear breakup determination must be performed on a pristine cornea. Plain fluorescein 0.125% is instilled into the lower cul-de-sac and, after several blinks, while the interpalpebral fissure is at a natural height, the corneal surface is scanned with a nonintense cobalt blue light. Dry spots occurring within 10 seconds are suggestive of KCS, but careful slit-lamp examination is necessary to identify other corneal pathologies that manifest in a rapid tear BUT (e.g., anterior membrane corneal dystrophy).

Measurement of tear production with Schirmer strips is useful but alone is not specific for pathological ocular dryness [3–6]. Schirmer strip testing can be done in various ways. The Schirmer II test for reflex tearing is uncommonly performed. The Schirmer I test, measuring total secretion, and the basal secretion Schirmer test, requiring topical anesthesia, are more commonly performed. The tear concentration of lysozyme, a normal product of the acinar and tubular cells of both the major and accessory lacrimal glands, falls as lacrimal gland tissue is progressively destroyed. Tear lysozyme level, as an individual test, has been shown to be a more sensitive indicator of Sjögren's syndrome than either the Schirmer I test or rose bengal staining [2, 7].

Tear lactoferrin levels are believed to function similarly to tear lysozyme as an indicator of lacrimal gland function and are useful in the diagnosis of KCS [8]. The lactoferrin immunological assay has the advantage of being an office diagnostic test with better specificity for KCS than either Schirmer testing or measurement of the tear film BUT. Tear osmolarity is elevated in aqueous-deficient states [9]. Testing requires a small volume of tears and measures the freezing point depression. Impression cytology of the bulbar conjunctiva of eyes with KCS displays squamous metaplasia with decreased or absent goblet cells and has developed as a means of grading the severity of KCS [10, 11]. Tear osmolarity and impression cytology may become the noninvasive, objective, reproducible criteria necessary for judging response to potential therapies. Most diagnoses of KCS are suspected on the basis of history and are confirmed with a clinical examination including slit-lamp examination with evaluation of tear BUT and rose bengal staining, and Schirmer testing.

■ Differential Diagnosis

Dry-eye syndrome is a feature of many systemic diseases. Aqueous tear deficiency is generally due to dysfunction, denervation, or infiltration and destruction of lacrimal gland tissue. Mucin deficiency is less common and results from vitamin A deficiency or conjunctival inflammation and scarring with destruction of goblet cells. Lipid abnormalities are usually due to meibomian gland dysfunction. The spectrum of these disorders is outlined in Table 1. Autoimmune and collagen vascular diseases comprise the bulk of this list, and the occurrence of dry eye in these diseases is not at all uncommon. Coll and associates [12] examined 78 patients with a variety of autoimmune disorders and found that 35% suffered from KCS as compared to 6% of a normal control group. Maintenance of the tear film is also dependent on a number of mechanical factors. The tear film normally undergoes evaporation and disruption and is reconstituted with each blink. Increasing the exposed tear film surface area will cause complications of desiccation, as will decreasing or abolishing the blink rate. In other instances, it is not a systemic disease that causes dry eye but rather a systemic medication.

Idiopathic Keratoconjunctivitis Sicca

The majority of patients with isolated dry-eye complaints have no major systemic disease to which the KCS can be attributed. Hence, routine extensive workup in the absence of systemic symptoms or signs is unwarranted. Menopausal or postmenopausal women are most commonly affected, from which an estrogen-dependent mechanism has been theorized but not proved [6]. Aqueous production decreases with increasing age and accounts for the prevalence of KCS in the elderly. Minor salivary gland biopsy in the elderly tends to show fibrosis and contracted lobules with a diffuse scattering of lymphocytes [13, 14] rather than the focal infiltration seen in Sjögren's syndrome.

Primary Sjögren's Syndrome

KCS in combination with mucosal dryness is referred to as the *sicca complex*. Difficulty chewing or ingesting dry foods is symptomatic of xerostomia. Xerostomia may increase the rate of dental caries. Upper airway dryness may cause a persistent cough or hoarseness. Vaginal dryness may lead to dyspareunia. Fox and colleagues [15] have proposed the following diagnostic criteria for Sjögren's syndrome: (1) objective evidence of KCS by rose bengal or fluorescein staining and decreased Schirmer's test (< 9 mm/5 min); (2) symptomatic xerostomia and decreased salivary flow rate; (3) serological evidence of an autoimmune process (e.g., positive rheumatoid factor, antinuclear antibody, Sjögren's syndrome antigen A [SS-A] or B [SS-B]); and (4) salivary gland histopathological confirmation showing at least two foci, each containing at least fifty lymphocytes, within a field of 4 mm^2. Nonuniformity of pathological involvement may result in apparent sampling errors. Since prior trauma or mucosal inflammation can cause nonspecific salivary gland lymphocytic infiltration, the lower-lip biopsy should be taken from an otherwise normal-appearing area. Progressive glandular destruction from lymphocytic infiltration and immune complex deposition occurs at an unpredictable pace.

Cases of primary Sjögren's syndrome developing immediately after infectious mononucleosis have been reported [16, 17]. Epstein-Barr virus (EBV) antigen has been found in lacrimal gland [17] and salivary gland [18] biopsy

Table 1 *Differential Diagnosis of Dry-Eye Syndrome*

- I. Aqueous deficiency
  - A. Idiopathic keratoconjunctivitis sicca
  - B. Sjögren's syndrome
    - 1. Primary Sjögren's syndrome
    - 2. Secondary Sjögren's syndrome
      - a. Classic
        - (1) Rheumatoid arthritis
        - (2) Systemic lupus erythematosus
        - (3) Systemic sclerosis
        - (4) Mixed connective tissue disease
        - (5) Relapsing polychondritis
        - (6) Wegener's granulomatosis
        - (7) Polyarteritis nodosa
        - (8) Hypergammaglobulinemic purpura of Waldenström
        - (9) Primary biliary cirrhosis
        - (10) Chronic active hepatitis
        - (11) Crohn's disease
      - b. Pseudo–Sjögren's syndrome
        - (1) Graft-versus-host disease
        - (2) Acquired immunodeficiency syndrome
  - C. Lacrimal gland infiltration
    - 1. Sarcoidosis
    - 2. Amyloidosis
    - 3. Systemic sclerosis
    - 4. Lymphoma
  - D. Miscellaneous
    - 1. Acne rosacea
    - 2. Multiple endocrine neoplasia IIb
  - E. Infectious diseases
    - 1. Infectious mononucleosis (Epstein-Barr virus)
    - 2. Lyme disease
  - F. Primary lacrimal gland dysfunction
    - 1. Congenital alacrima
    - 2. Anhidrotic ectodermal dysplasia
  - G. Lacrimal gland denervation
    - 1. Congenital
      - a. Familial dysautonomia (Riley-Day syndrome)
      - b. Möbius syndrome
    - 2. Adult-onset: adult dysautonomia (Shy-Drager syndrome)
    - 3. Mechanical
      - a. Brainstem lesions
      - b. Cerebellopontine angle tumors
      - c. Middle fossa floor lesions
      - d. Posterolateral orbit wall fracture (zygomaticotemporal nerve)
    - 4. Chemical
      - a. Botulism intoxication
      - b. Medication-induced
- II. Mucin deficiency
  - A. Nutritional deficiency: hypovitaminosis A
  - B. Conjunctival inflammation and scarring
    - 1. Cicatricial pemphigoid
    - 2. Erythema multiforme (Stevens-Johnson syndrome)

continued

Table 1 *(continued)*

3. Toxic epidermal necrolysis
4. Graft-versus-host disease
C. Miscellaneous: familial dysautonomia
III. Lipid abnormality
A. Acne rosacea
B. Anhidrotic ectodermal dysplasia—lipid deficiency
IV. Exposure
A. Proptosis: thyroid disorders
B. Decreased or absent blink rate: parkinsonism

in some patients with primary Sjögren's syndrome. It is hypothesized that in predisposed (e.g., HLA type) individuals, EBV infection may cause glandular disease through either persistent viral activation or reactivation. Cytomegalovirus and adenovirus infections have also been proposed as possible etiological factors [19, 20].

Primary Sjögren's syndrome may manifest with a generalized fatigue or depression. Systemic involvement may result in central and peripheral nervous system disease, pneumonitis, vasculitis, renal disease, arthralgias, and myositis. Ocular disease other than KCS may include uveitis, optic neuritis, and retinal vasculitis.

In patients with primary Sjögren's syndrome, HLA-B8 and HLA-DRw3 histocompatibility antigens are significantly more common [21]. Serum tests for autoantibodies to SS-A (Ro) and SS-B (La) support the diagnosis of Sjögren's syndrome [22]. Although lacrimal gland biopsy would be confirmatory, some regard accessory salivary gland biopsy through a labial incision as a more benign procedure.

Sjögren's syndrome existing as a component of another identifiable autoimmune disease is designated *secondary Sjögren's syndrome.*

Rheumatoid Arthritis

Rheumatoid arthritis (RA) is a chronic inflammatory, multisystem, immunologically mediated disease of unknown etiology. Diagnosis requires confirmation of seven of the following eleven criteria: (1) morning stiffness; (2) pain on motion or tenderness in at least one joint; (3) swelling in at least one joint; (4) swelling of at least one other joint; (5) symmetrical joint swelling; (6) subcutaneous nodules; (7) roentgenographic changes; (8) positive rheumatoid factor; (9) poor mucin precipitate from synovial fluid; (10) characteristic histological changes in synovium; and (11) characteristic histological changes in a nodule [23].

Approximately 1% of the population is affected, with onset most commonly in the fourth to fifth decade of life. Women are two to three times more commonly affected than men [24]. There appear to be predisposing genetic and environmental factors. Rheumatoid factor, an IgM immunoglobulin–binding IgG, although found in more than 70% of RA patients, may also be found in 5% of the normal population and in 10 to 20% of individuals older than 65 years. An extensive list of other conditions is also associated with a positive rheumatoid factor. A high rheumatoid factor titer, however, is noteworthy because it is believed to be prognostic of severe and extraarticular disease.

Ocular complications in RA include KCS, peripheral corneal infiltrates, sterile corneal ulceration, episcleritis, scleritis, uveitis, and extraocular myositis [25]. In a study from Greece, although only 18% of 111 patients with RA had subjective complaints of dry eyes, 34 patients met histopathological criteria for the diagnosis of Sjögren's syndrome. Rose bengal staining was observed in 58 patients, and 50 had abnormal Schirmer I test results [26].

Systemic Lupus Erythematosus

Systemic lupus erythematosus (SLE) is a chronic inflammatory, immunologically mediated disease of unknown etiology, the pathogenesis of which involves poorly regulated production of various antibodies and immune complexes. Diagnosis is based on meeting four of eleven criteria: (1) malar rash; (2) discoid rash; (3) cutaneous photosensitivity; (4) oral ulcers; (5) nonerosive polyarthritis; (6) pleurisy, pericarditis, or myocarditis; (7) proteinuria or glomerulonephritis; (8) seizures or psychosis; (9) hemolytic anemia, leukopenia, or thrombocytopenia; (10) antibodies to double-stranded DNA (anti-dsDNA) or smooth-muscle antigen (anti-Sm), or false-positive syphilis serology (VDRL); and (11) non-drug-induced antinuclear antibodies (ANA). The false-positive syphilis serology is due to antibodies to the phospholipid cardiolipin. Adolescent and young women are affected approximately eight times as often as men [27].

KCS is the most common ocular finding, occurring in 7 to 54% of patients [28–30]. Spaeth [31] found that 87% of the SLE patients he examined had fluorescein corneal staining. The presence of anti-Ro and anti-La autoantibodies has been correlated with up to a 49% incidence of KCS and with a reduced frequency of renal disease [32]. Conjunctivitis, episcleritis, keratitis (epithelial, interstitial, and ulcerative), uveitis, retinal vasculitis, and optic neuritis can occur.

Systemic Sclerosis

Systemic sclerosis or scleroderma is a generalized disorder of unknown etiology characterized by fibrosis and degenerative changes in the skin, synovium, small arteries, and internal organs including the esophagus, intestine, lungs, heart, kidney, and thyroid. Women are affected three to four times as often as men [23]. Environmental factors have been associated.

For most patients, the initial complaint is either Raynaud's phenomenon or thickening and tightening of the skin of the fingers. Scleroderma may manifest as a diffuse cutaneous form with a greater likelihood of subsequent visceral disease or as a less severe limited cutaneous form displaying features of CREST syndrome. *CREST* is an acronym for *c*alcinosis, *R*aynaud's phenomenon, *e*sophageal dysmotility, *s*clerodactyly, and *t*elangiectasis.

Overproduction of normal collagen results in fibrosis. Histopathological evaluation of salivary gland biopsies taken from systemic sclerosis patients with sicca complex may reveal the characteristic lymphocytic infiltrates of Sjögren's syndrome or the fibrosis of scleroderma [33]. Serum antibodies to SS-A (Ro) or SS-B (La) are found in patients with lymphocytic infiltrations but not in patients with glandular fibrosis. As many as 25% of patients develop KCS, whereas 20% of patients are diagnosed as having secondary Sjögren's syndrome [33–35].

Mixed Connective Tissue Disease

Mixed connective tissue disease (MCTD) is characterized by clinical features of RA, SLE, systemic sclerosis, and polymyositis. The typical findings consist of Raynaud's phenomenon, polyarthralgia or arthritis, esophageal hypomotility, diminished pulmonary diffusing capacity, and inflammatory myopathy. The disease affects women four times more frequently than men. The age range extends from 4 to 80 years, with a mean of 37 years [23]. Serological characteristics in most patients include a high-titer ANA ($\geq$ 1:1,000) in a speckled pattern and a high titer of circulating antibody to a ribonuclease-sensitive nuclear ribonucleoprotein component of extractable nuclear antigen (ENA). KCS is found in approximately 36% of patients [36].

Relapsing Polychondritis

Relapsing polychondritis is a rare disease characterized by episodic inflammation and destruction of cartilage. It can be associated with a systemic vasculitis and cardiopulmonary involvement. A diagnosis is based on clinical findings including recurrent chondritis of the auricles, ocular inflammation, chondritis of the laryngeal or tracheal cartilage, and cochlear or vestibular damage manifested by neurosensory hearing loss, tinnitus, or vertigo. Ocular findings occur in 60% of patients and include KCS, conjunctivitis, episcleritis, scleritis, corneal melts, uveitis, optic neuritis, periorbital edema, and extraocular muscle palsies [37].

Wegener's Granulomatosis

Wegener's granulomatosis is a systemic vasculitis characterized by granuloma formation in the respiratory tract, necrotizing glomerulonephritis, and a disseminated vasculitis affecting both arteries and veins. More than 90% of patients have upper respiratory tract (sinus) involvement [38]. Diagnosis is made on finding histopathological evidence of a necrotizing granulomatous vasculitis in the clinical setting of upper and lower respiratory tract disease and glomerulonephritis. Antineutrophil cytoplasmic antibodies (ANCA) are 100% sensitive and 88% specific for active Wegener's granulomatosis [39]. Ocular signs develop in 28 to 40% of patients and include proptosis, KCS, conjunctivitis, episcleritis, scleritis, corneal ulceration, uveitis, retinal vasculitis, extraocular muscle palsies, and optic nerve disease [40, 41]. The incidence of KCS was 29% in one series [42]. Untreated, Wegener's granulomatosis is fatal. Systemic corticosteroids and cyclophosphamide achieve long-term remission in more than 90% of patients [43].

Polyarteritis Nodosa

Polyarteritis nodosa (PAN) produces a necrotizing vasculitis of small and medium arteries. Characteristically, renal and visceral arteries are involved and pulmonary arteries are spared. Diagnosis is based on biopsy. Thirty percent of patients may have a hepatitis B antigenemia. ANCA titers have a sensitivity of 80% and a specificity of 88% [39]. Aside from KCS, PAN has been associated with inflammatory processes involving virtually every ocular structure. Cogan's syndrome may be a limited form of PAN.

Benign Hypergammaglobulinemic Purpura of Waldenström

Waldenström [44] described this syndrome of recurrent purpura of the lower extremities, increased erythrocyte sedimentation rate, mild anemia, and hypergammaglobulinemia in 1943. The disorder may be primary or associated with other disorders including SLE, polymyositis, RA, and sarcoidosis. The incidence in women is four times that in men. The hypergammaglobulinemia has a heterogeneous pattern like that seen in SLE. Circulating immune complexes localize in the skin as intradermal deposits. As many as 50% of cases are complicated by symptoms and features of Sjögren's syndrome, leading some to regard these diseases as within a common continuum varying only in the most prominent clinical manifestation [45, 46].

Liver Disease

Primary biliary cirrhosis, postnecrotic cirrhosis, and chronic active hepatitis are liver disorders associated with hyperglobulinemia and non-organ-specific autoantibodies. Primary biliary cirrhosis is a chronic progressive disease primarily affecting young to middle-aged women. It is frequently associated with a variety of autoimmune disorders, particularly systemic sclerosis, thyroiditis, rheumatoid arthritis, and Sjögren's syndrome. Although many patients are asymptomatic, symptoms may include pruritus, hyperpigmentation, jaundice, and hepatosplenomegaly. Elevation of the serum alkaline phosphatase level during routine screening may lead to the diagnosis of presymptomatic or asymptomatic patients. Serum IgG antimitochondrial antibodies, found in more than 95% of patients, support the diagnosis. Histopathologically, there is a nonsuppurative destructive cholangitis. The incidence of KCS is reported as varying from 36 to 72% [47, 48]. Hansen and colleagues [49] found lymphocytic infiltrates typical of Sjögren's syndrome in 14 of 15 biopsies of minor salivary glands from patients with primary biliary cirrhosis. Malabsorption of vitamin A secondary to impaired bile excretion can lead to hypovitaminosis A, a cause of both night blindness and dry eyes.

Chronic active hepatitis and postnecrotic cirrhosis are most frequently associated with a history of viral hepatitis. Approximately 20% of patients have positive serological tests for hepatitis B surface antigen (HB_sAg) [48]. Exposure to a variety of toxins has also been linked to these disorders. Histopathologically, chronic active hepatitis is characterized by ongoing hepatic necrosis and inflammation. In end-stage disease (i.e., postnecrotic cirrhosis), the liver appears shrunken and scarred. Sicca complex has been found in 40% of patients [47].

Graft-Versus-Host Disease

Graft-versus-host disease (GVHD) is a major complication following allogeneic bone marrow transplantation. It occurs when immunologically competent donor cells, presumably T lymphocytes, react against the host. Clinical features are skin rash, hepatitis, diarrhea, and lymphopenia. GVHD frequently leads to major impairment of target organs and often has a fatal outcome.

Reported ocular complications of GVHD include conjunctivitis, corneal ulceration, iridocyclitis, and choroiditis [50]. KCS, found in up to 62% of patients, is the most frequently noted complication [50–54]. Lacrimal gland biopsies show differing histopathological features at different stages of the disease. Franklin and co-workers [50], in a series of patients with early-onset GVHD (prior to 150 days posttransplant) found epithelial cell flattening and inspissation of ducts without inflammatory cell infiltrates. In later-onset disease, a prominent lymphocytic infiltrate characteristic of Sjögren's syndrome has been observed [54].

Acquired Immune Deficiency Syndrome

Acquired immune deficiency syndrome (AIDS) is caused by infection with the human immunodeficiency virus type 1 (HIV-1). The syndrome is defined as the occurrence of life-threatening opportunistic infections or Kaposi's sarcoma in a person with no other underlying immunosuppressive disease and who has not received immunosuppressive therapy. Ophthalmic complications include KCS, cotton-wool spots, cytomegalovirus and *Pneumocystis carinii* retinitis, syphilitic and tuberculous uveitis, and cryptococcal choroiditis. KCS occurs in 21% of patients with HIV-1 infection [55] and in up to 50% of patients with AIDS [56]. Histopathological examination of biopsy specimens from minor salivary glands in patients with the sicca complex shows lymphocytic infiltration of the glandular parenchyma typical of Sjögren's syndrome [57].

Sarcoidosis

Sarcoidosis is a multisystem disease characterized by noncaseating granulomatous inflammation. The disease initially presents between the third and fifth decades of life. Women are affected slightly more commonly than men. The most common findings are bilateral hilar adenopathy, pulmonary infiltrates, and skin and eye lesions. In the absence of confirmatory histopathology, a presumptive diagnosis can be supported by an elevated serum angiotensin-converting enzyme (ACE) and a positive gallium scan. KCS, conjunctival granulomas, and uveitis are the most common ocular manifestations, although almost any ocular structure may ultimately become involved [58, 59]. Salivary or lacrimal gland biopsy may differentiate sarcoidosis from Sjögren's syndrome. Drosos and colleagues [60] reviewed biopsies of minor salivary glands in 5 patients with sarcoidosis and apparent secondary Sjögren's syndrome and found noncaseating granulomas in 3 specimens and lymphocytic infiltrates in the other 2. Tear lysozyme, normally lowered in Sjögren's syndrome, may be elevated due to macrophage and giant cell activity within lacrimal gland granulomas [61]. Karma [62] found conjunctival granulomas to be the most common ophthalmic finding. A noncaseating granuloma seen on biopsy of one of these yellowish golden fleshy nodules in a patient with KCS is diagnostic.

Amyloidosis

Amyloidosis is characterized by the deposition of a noninflammatory, extracellular, amorphous, eosinophilic protein—amyloid. Among the numerous biochemical and associated clinical forms of amyloid are (1) amyloid light chain (AL), homologous to the *N*-terminal region of the variable fragment of an immunoglobulin light chain, in primary systemic and multiple myeloma–associated amyloid; (2) AA protein in amyloid secondary to chronic infections, inflammatory disorders, and neoplasms; (3) AF protein (prealbumin) in familial amyloid polyneuropathy; (4) AE protein (precalcitonin) in medullary carcinoma of the thyroid; (5) A4 protein in Alzheimer's disease; and (6) $beta_2$-microglobulin in chronic hemodialysis.

Clinical manifestations vary with the organ system involved. Histopathological evidence of amyloid deposition in minor salivary glands has been correlated with the sicca complex [63] but appears to be a relatively rare manifestation of amyloidosis. Any ocular structure may be involved. Systemic amyloidosis is slowly progressive with variable survival. Definitive therapy is lacking, but colchicine has shown promise.

Erythema Multiforme and Toxic Epidermal Necrolysis

Erythema multiforme and toxic epidermal necrolysis (Lyell's disease) are blistering dermatological disorders that may involve the conjunctivae and eyelids. The skin lesions of erythema multiforme are pink-red macules and edematous papules, often with central vesiculation, or petechiae formation giving an iris or bull's-eye appearance. Distribution is generally symmetrical, involving the extensor areas of the limbs, palms, soles, and mucous membranes. Preceding or concurrent fever and malaise are common. Stevens-Johnson syndrome is a severe variant in which the mucous membranes are predominantly involved. Erythema multiforme has been associated with drugs (e.g., barbiturates, sulfonamides); bacterial, fungal, and viral infections; vaccinations; radiation therapy; environmental toxins; and various systemic diseases. Dermal inflammation typifies erythema multiforme, and bullae contain exudate from dermal vessels and polymorphic cellular debris.

Toxic epidermal necrolysis is characterized by more flaccid skin bullae. Mechanical epidermolysis (Nikolsky's sign) may precede blister formation. The Nikolsky sign, which helps to distinguish toxic epidermal necrolysis from erythema multiforme, is found in other bullous skin diseases such as staphylococcal scalded skin syndrome (SSSS). However, in toxic epidermal necrolysis cleavage occurs at the basal cell layer, whereas cleavage occurs within the epidermis in SSSS.

The principal ocular manifestation of both illnesses is a conjunctivitis, which may be catarrhal, purulent, or pseudomembranous [64–66]. Topical or systemic corticosteroids together with mechanical disruption or prevention of conjunctival adhesions early in the acute stages may minimize the destructive scarification. Long-term complications include ectropion, entropion, trichiasis, conjunctival cicatrization and symblepharon formation, corneal scarring, and ulceration. KCS occurs secondary to scarring of the orifices of the aqueous and lipid-secreting glands supplying the tear film and to destruction of conjunctival goblet cells, with a resulting mucin deficiency [66].

Cicatricial Pemphigoid

Cicatricial pemphigoid (benign mucous membrane pemphigoid) is a chronic disabling inflammatory disease characterized by bullae or erosions affecting mucous membranes more commonly than skin. Nonocular complications include posterior nasal stricture, laryngeal scarring, esophageal stricture, and urethral stenosis. Ocular cicatricial pemphigoid occurred in 77% of patients in one study [67]. Diagnosis is made by finding immunoglobulin and complement deposition along the conjunctival basement membrane zone. If untreated, the course is progressive and characterized by refractory conjunctivitis, forniceal shrinkage, symblepharon formation, entropion, trichiasis and, ultimately, corneal opacification and possible ulceration. KCS occurs secondary to occlusion of the aqueous and lipid-secreting glands by scar tissue, complicated by goblet cell dropout [68]. Dapsone is frequently used as first-line therapy. Cyclophosphamide with or without systemic corticosteroids is reserved for refractory or severe, rapidly progressive disease.

Acne Rosacea

Acne rosacea is characterized by erythema and multiple telangiectases over the nose, cheeks, forehead, and chin. Acneiform lesions and chronic hypertrophy of the facial sebaceous glands are found in the more severe cases. Chronic blepharitis is the most frequent ocular abnormality. Other ocular problems include meibomianitis, styes, chalazia, papillary conjunctivitis, episcleritis, keratoconjunctivitis, KCS, and ulcerative keratitis. The symptoms of chronic blepharitis may be similar to those of keratitis sicca. Decreased tear production was observed in 36% of patients followed by Lemp and colleagues [69], and treatment with tetracycline did not improve aqueous tear production.

Multiple Sclerosis

Multiple sclerosis (MS) is a demyelinating disease of the central nervous system presenting commonly to ophthalmologists as retrobulbar optic neuritis and, less commonly, as a pars planitis. Alexander and associates [70] found that 20 of 200 patients with primary Sjögren's syndrome had central nervous system manifestations mimicking MS. Each of these patients satisfied accepted clinical criteria for the diagnosis of MS. Many of the patients appeared to stabilize or improve when treated with corticosteroids.

A high incidence of keratitis sicca has been found in the MS population. In two studies, the frequency appeared to be between 33 and 42% of patients [71, 72].

Dysautonomic Syndromes

Familial dysautonomia (Riley-Day syndrome) is an autosomal recessive congenital disorder of autonomic homeostasis and sensory appreciation [73–75]. The disorder is limited almost entirely to children of Ashkenazic Jewish ancestry [76]. Systemic manifestations include abnormal swallowing reflex, labile blood pressure, labile body temperature, hypotonia, and developmental delay. A pathognomonic feature is the absence of fungiform papillae and taste buds on the tongue. Ocular complications are due to decreased lacrimation and corneal hypoesthesia. Ocular findings include myopia, convergence insufficiency, exodeviations, Adie's pupil, blepharitis, retinal vascular tortuosity, and optic neuropathy. Although parent education and cooperation may reduce the need for it, tarsorrhaphy may be required to prevent corneal ulceration and permanent scarring.

Adult dysautonomia (Shy-Drager syndrome) is a progressive degenerative disorder of the central nervous system and, occasionally, of the peripheral nervous system and is of unknown etiology. Autonomic dysfunction may result in postural hypotension, urinary bladder dysfunction, constipation, impotence, pupillary asymmetry, and partial Horner's syndrome. Extrapyramidal dysfunction may produce parkinsonian manifestations. Complaints of xerophthalmia and xerostomia are common [77].

Anhidrotic Ectodermal Dysplasia

Anhidrotic ectodermal dysplasia is a sex-linked recessive disease characterized by absence of eccrine sweating and an unusual facies. At birth, affected infants appear normal, but by 1 year of age the disease is generally manifest. The head displays a square forehead, prominent frontal bossing and supraorbital ridges, depression of the central face, a pointed nose and chin, and sparse facial and scalp hair. Ocular findings include KCS, increased periorbital pigmentation, mongoloid slant to the eyelids, absence of eyebrows and lashes, stenosis of the inferior puncta, corneal opacities, iris and pupillary abnormalities, and congenital cataracts [78].

Congenital Alacrima

Bilateral congenital absence of tears is usually related to familial dysautonomia or anhidrotic ectodermal dysplasia. It may also be seen in the Möbius syndrome. Unilateral cases of unknown etiology have been observed in otherwise normal infants. Ocular findings in these cases span from mild KCS to keratinization of the corneal and conjunctival surfaces [79].

Botulism

Botulism intoxication is due to ingestion of a toxin produced by *Clostridium botulinum.* Eight toxins (A through G) have been identified, but A, B, and E are of most clinical importance. Type A toxin disease is characterized by paralysis and frequently death within 18 to 36 hours after eating contaminated food.

In contrast, type B contamination produces non-life-threatening autonomic dysfunction including constipation, orthostatic dizziness, impaired micturition, and sexual dysfunction. Konig and colleagues [80] found a 100% incidence of dry-eye and dry-mouth complaints in a series of 9 patients, with symptoms persisting for months. Guanidine hydrochloride, taken orally, provided anecdotal relief.

Multiple Endocrine Neoplasia

Multiple endocrine neoplasia (MEN) has two major subgroups. MEN-I (Wermer's syndrome) includes neoplasia or hyperplasia of the pituitary, pancreas, and parathyroid glands. MEN-II is characterized by the presence of medullary carcinoma of the thyroid, pheochromocytoma, and hyperparathyroidism. MEN-IIa (Sipple's syndrome) is phenotypically normal, whereas MEN-IIb is characterized by a marfanoid habitus and thickened eyelids, lips, and tongue due to mucosal neuromas. Dry eye, a prominent feature of MEN-IIb, occurs in two-thirds of patients. The pathophysiology is unknown [81]. MEN-IIb is better known to ophthalmologists in the differential diagnosis of prominent corneal nerves.

Hypovitaminosis A

Vitamin A dietary deficiency is a major cause of childhood blindness and an important public health problem in developing nations. Sommer and Sugana [82] have reported that, in Asia alone, 5 million children are affected by xerophthalmia every year. The earliest changes observed clinically are a punctate keratopathy and dry patches on the bulbar conjunctiva [83, 84]. Persistent vitamin A deficiency results in corneal and conjunctival xerosis, Bitot's spots, corneal ulceration, and keratomalacia [85]. Rose bengal staining demonstrates spotty interpalpebral epithelial injury secondary to desiccation. These findings correlate histopathologically with loss of mucin-secreting goblet cells and squamous metaplasia of epithelial cells [85, 86].

Bitot's spots are raised, compact, refractile, conjunctival lesions with a silvery gray hue and a foamy surface. They are not pathognomonic of vitamin A deficiency. When scraped off with a spatula, the keratinized debris is not infrequently colonized by *Corynebacterium xerosis.* These bacteria are not believed to play an etiological role.

Measles, a not uncommon childhood viral exanthem, may precipitously decompensate an eye with xerosis into keratomalacia and ensuing complications. Keratomalacia is a characteristic necrosis of the entire thickness of the cornea without significant inflammatory cell infiltration. These corneal ulcers often become secondarily infected, perforate, and result in endophthalmitis or secondary angle closure glaucoma.

Ocular dryness in vitamin A deficiency is due to mucin deficiency, which in turn produces an unstable precorneal tear film [87]. Mucin deficiency is the result of conjunctival goblet cell loss, which can be monitored by conjunctival impression cytology [85]. Recording the tear film BUT, which is expected to be markedly abbreviated, can be useful [84]. There may be an associated aqueous deficiency. Dark adaptation is the most sensitive test for vitamin A deficiency. Adequate food intake and incorporating leafy vegetables into the diet would prevent this disease.

Hypovitaminosis A in the presence of an adequate diet may be related to disorders of digestion, absorption, transport, storage, and metabolism [84]. Malabsorption of vitamin A and other fat-soluble vitamins can occur in chronic pancreatitis, chronic liver disease, alcoholism, and cystic fibrosis, after gastrectomy or small bowel resection, and in various other intestinal diseases. A failure in transport of vitamin A occurs in abetalipoproteinemia.

Brainstem and Cranial Nerve Lesions

Tear secretion is neurologically modulated via interactions of the trigeminal, facial, and cervical sympathetic fibers. The afferent path is primarily the lacrimal nerve, a tributary of the ophthalmic division of the fifth nerve. The efferent pathway begins in the pontine tegmentum above the superior salivary nucleus. These seventh nerve fibers travel through the nervus intermedius, pass through the facial (geniculate) ganglion and greater superficial petrosal nerve (lateral to the trigeminal ganglion in the floor of the middle fossa), join the deep petrosal nerve to form the vidian nerve, and synapse in the sphenopalatine ganglion. Postganglionic neurons course through the zygomatic nerve after leaving the trigeminal ganglion. Preganglionic sympathetic fibers from the hypothalamus lead to postganglionic sympathetic fibers originating in the superior cervical ganglion or carotid plexus, which in turn find their way to the lacrimal gland along the lacrimal artery or lacrimal nerve.

Rare instances of reduced tear secretion have been observed in patients with brainstem lesions [88]. These lesions appear to involve the lacrimal nucleus and are associated with other signs of brainstem dysfunction.

Lesions in the cerebellopontine angle and internal auditory meatus can interrupt fibers of the nervus intermedius carrying innervation to the lacrimal gland. Acoustic neuromas are most common in this region and may cause hearing loss, vestibular palsy, facial palsy, loss of taste, hyperacusis, and decreased lacrimation. Lesions in the floor of the middle fossa (e.g., nasopharyngeal carcinoma, meningioma) injuring the superficial petrosal nerve may cause decreased lacrimation (associated with sixth nerve palsy) and facial pain or numbness. Aneurysms of the carotid artery and traumatic fractures can also injure this nerve. Injury to the zygomaticotemporal nerve, often the result of a fracture of the posterior lateral wall of the orbit, produces postganglionic denervation of the lacrimal gland [88].

Reduced ocular surface sensation can decrease tear secretion by 60 to 75%. Experimental trigeminal ganglion lesions in rabbits have been associated with an increased tear osmolarity, rose bengal staining, decreased goblet cell density, and conjunctival epithelial cell metaplasia [89].

Thyroid Disorders

Complications of corneal exposure occur through a number of mechanisms. Nocturnal lagophthalmos, reduced blink rate, and increased interpalpebral fissure height with or without proptosis all lead to corneal and conjunctival desiccation.

Parkinsonism

Parkinson's disease and drug-induced parkinsonism have a typical clinical picture that includes stooped posture, stiffness and slowness of movement, fixity of facial expression, and rhythmic tremor of the limbs that may subside on willed movement and relaxation. Biochemically, dopaminergic insufficiency or blockade in the nigrostriatal pathway has been shown to be responsible. The disorder typically begins asymmetrically, with a slight tremor in a hand or leg. A general hypokinesia and stiffness in the musculature is also apparent at an early stage. A staring and immobile facial expression may be recognized. Tremor may be minimal but can be recognized in the hands, legs, lips, tongue, neck muscles, and eyelids when they are gently closed. Myerson's sign, an inability to suppress blinking following tapping on the nasion, is common.

Table 2 *Drugs Associated with Decreased Lacrimation*

Acebutolol	Disopyramide	Opium
Acetophenazine	Doxylamine	Oxprenolol
Albuterol	Dronabinol	Perazine
Aluminum nicotinate	Ether	Periciazine
Amitriptyline	Ethopropazine	Perphenazine
Antazoline	Etretinate	Pheniramine
Atenolol	Fluphenazine	Pimozide
Atropine	Hashish	Pindolol
Azatadine	Hexamethonium	Piperacetazine
Belladonna	Homatropine	Polythiazide
Bendroflumethazide	Hydrochlorothiazide	Practolol
Benzalkonium	Hydroflumethazide	Prochlorperazine
Benzthiazide	Imipramine	Promazine
Brompheniramine	Indapamide	Promethazine
Busulfan	Isotretinoin	Propiomazine
Butaperazine	Labetolol	Propranolol
Carbinoxamine	Marijuana	Protriptyline
Carphenazine	Mesoridazine	Pyrilamine
Chlorisondamine	Methdilazine	Quinethazone
Chlorothiazide	Methotrexate	Scopolamine
Chlorpheniramine	Methotrimeprazine	Tetrahydrocannabinol (THC)
Chlorpromazine	Methoxsalen	Thiethylperazine
Chlorthalidone	Methscopolamine	Thiopropazate
Cimetidine	Methyclothiazide	Thioproperazine
Clemastine	Methyldopa	Thioridazine
Clonidine	Methylthiouracil	Timolol
Cyclothiazide	Metolazone	Trichlormethiazide
Cyproheptadine	Metoprolol	Trichloroethylene
Desipramine	Morphine	Trifluoperazine
Dexbrompheniramine	Nadolol	Triflupromazine
Dexchlorpheniramine	Niacin	Trimeprazine
Diethazine	Niacinamide	Trioxsalen
Dimethindene	Nicotinyl alcohol	Tripelennamine
Diphenhydramine	Nitrous oxide	Triprolidine
Diphenylpyraline	Nortriptyline	

Source: From Fraunfelder FT, Decreased lacrimation. In: Fraunfelder FT, ed. Drug-induced ocular side effects and drug interactions. Philadelphia: Lea & Febiger, 1989:513–514.

Seborrhea, which is frequently seen, may lead to recurrent hordeola and blepharitis. A reduced frequency of blinking may cause dry-eye problems. Other ocular manifestations of parkinsonism are decreased convergence, limited upgaze, hypometric saccades, and oculogyric crises [90].

Drug-Related Dry-Eye Syndrome

Numerous medications have been associated with dry-eye syndrome, as listed in Table 2 [91].

■ Treatment of Dry Eye

Ocular lubricants, including artificial tear drops and ointments, relieve dry-eye symptoms and signs of KCS in the majority of patients with mild to moderate disease. Medicamentosa (toxic keratoconjunctivitis) is more common in dry-eye patients and requires the discontinuation of preserved artificial lubricants. When frequent instillation of preservative-free lubricants is required, the patient generally will benefit from some form of punctal occlusion to utilize their own natural tear production maximally. Use of a mucolytic, such as 10 or 20% acetylcysteine four to five times daily, can be helpful [92]. Other options available to the patient include moisture chambers, room humidifiers, and tarsorrhaphy.

■ Comments

A wide variety of systemic illnesses are associated with the dry-eye syndrome. Early diagnosis of many of these conditions and appropriate intervention can drastically change outcome. Mortality as well as ocular and systemic morbidity can be reduced. It is the challenge of the astute physician to recognize the sometimes subtle signs of an underlying systemic disease and to direct the patient appropriately for further evaluation and treatment.

This work was supported in part by an unrestricted grant from Research to Prevent Blindness, Inc., New York, NY.

■ References

1. Sjögren H, Bloch KJ. Keratoconjunctivitis sicca and the Sjögren syndrome. Surv Ophthalmol 1971;16:145–159
2. van Bijsterveld OP. Diagnostic tests in the sicca syndrome. Arch Ophthalmol 1969;82:10–14
3. Henderson JW, Prough WA. Influence of age and sex on tears. Arch Ophthalmol 1950;43:224–231
4. DeRötth AFM. On the hypofunction of the lacrimal gland. Am J Ophthalmol 1941;24:20–25
5. Lamberts DW. Dry eye and tear deficiency. Int Ophthalmol Clin 1983;23:123–130

6. DeRötth AFM. Low flow of tears—the dry eye. Am J Ophthalmol 1952;35: 782–787
7. Regan E. The lysozyme content of tears. Am J Ophthalmol 1950;33:600–605
8. Goren MB, Goren SB. Diagnostic tests in patients with symptoms of keratoconjunctivitis sicca. Am J Ophthalmol 1988;106:570–574
9. Gilbard JP, Farris RL, Santamaria J. Osmolarity of tear microvolumes in keratoconjunctivitis sicca. Arch Ophthalmol 1978;96:677–681
10. Nelson JD, Havener VR, Cameron JD. Cellulose acetate impressions of the ocular surface. Arch Ophthalmol 1983;101:1869–1872
11. Tseng SCG. Staging of conjunctival squamous metaplasia by impression cytology. Ophthalmology 1985;92:728–733
12. Coll J, Rives A, Grino MC, et al. Prevalence of Sjögren's syndrome in autoimmune diseases. Ann Rheum Dis 1987;46:286–289
13. Waterhouse J, Doniach D. Postmortem prevalence of focal lymphocytic adenitis of the submandibular gland. J Pathol 1986;91:53–81
14. Chisholm D, Waterhouse J, Mason D. Lymphocytic sialadenitis in the major and minor glands; a correlation in postmortem subjects. J Clin Pathol 1970;23:690–694
15. Fox RI, Robinson CA, Curd JG, et al. Sjögren's syndrome: proposed criteria for classification. Arthritis Rheum 1986;29:577–585
16. Whittingham S, McNeilage LJ, Mackay IR. Epstein-Barr virus as an etiological agent in primary Sjögren's syndrome. Med Hypotheses 1987;22:373–386
17. Pflugfelder SC, Tseng SCG, Pepose JS, et al. Epstein-Barr virus infection and immunologic dysfunction in patients with aqueous tear deficiency. Ophthalmology 1990;97:313–323
18. Fox RI, Pearson G, Vaughan JH. Detection of Epstein-Barr virus–associated antigens and DNA in salivary gland biopsies from patients with Sjögren's syndrome. J Immunol 1986;137:3162–3168
19. Shillitoe EJ, Daniels TE, Whitcher JP, et al. Antibody to cytomegalovirus in patients with Sjögren's syndrome. Arthritis Rheum 1982;25:260–265
20. Rosa MA, Gottlieb E, Lerner MR, Steitz JA. Autoantibodies to small nuclear ribonucleoproteins. A strong association between anti-SS-B(La), HLA-B8 and primary Sjögren's syndrome. Mol Cell Biol 1981;1:785
21. Fye KH, Terasaki PI, Michalski JP, et al. Relationship of HLA-Dw3 and HLA-B8 to Sjögren's syndrome. Arthritis Rheum 1978;21:337–339
22. Reichlin M. Significance of the Ro antigen system. J Clin Immunol 1986;6:339–348
23. Rodnan GP, Schumacher HR, eds. Primer on the rheumatic diseases. Atlanta: Arthritis Foundation, 1983
24. Lipsky PE. Rheumatoid arthritis. In: Wilson JD, Braunwald E, Isselbacher KJ, et al, eds. Harrison's principles of internal medicine. New York: McGraw-Hill, 1991:1437–1443
25. Whitson WE, Krachmer JH. Adult rheumatoid arthritis. In: Gold DH, Weingeist T, eds. The eye in systemic disease. Philadelphia: Lippincott, 1990:61–64
26. Andonopoulos AP, Drosos AA, Skopouli FN, et al. Secondary Sjögren's syndrome in rheumatoid arthritis. J Rheumatol 1987;14:1098–1103
27. Hahn BH. Systemic lupus erythematosus. In: Wilson JD, Braunwald E, Isselbacher KJ, et al, eds. Harrison's principles of internal medicine. New York: McGraw-Hill, 1991:1432–1437
28. Grennan DM, Forrester J. Involvement of the eye in SLE and scleroderma. Ann Rheum Dis 1977;36:152–156
29. Alarcon-Segovia D, Ibanez G, Velazquez-Forero F, et al. Sjögren's syndrome in systemic lupus erythematosus. Ann Intern Med 1974;81:577–583
30. Andonopoulos AP, Skopouli FN, Dimou GS, et al. Sjögren's syndrome in systemic lupus erythematosus. J Rheumatol 1990;17:201–204

31. Spaeth GL. Corneal staining in systemic lupus erythematosus. N Engl J Med 1967;276:1168–1171
32. Maddison PJ, Isenberg DA, Goulding NJ, et al. Anti La (SSB) identifies a distinctive subgroup of systemic lupus erythematosus. Br J Rheumatol 1988;27:27–31
33. Drosos AA, Andonopoulos AP, Costopoulos JS, et al. Sjögren's syndrome in progressive systemic sclerosis. J Rheumatol 1988;15:965–968
34. West RH, Barnett AJ. Ocular involvement in scleroderma. Br J Ophthalmol 1979;63:845–847
35. Horan EC. Ophthalmic manifestations of progressive systemic sclerosis. Br J Ophthalmol 1969;53:388–392
36. Alarcon-Segovia D. Symptomatic Sjögren's syndrome in mixed connective tissue disease. J Rheumatol 1976;3:191–195
37. Isaak BL, Liesegang TJ, Michet CJ. Ocular and systemic findings in relapsing polychondritis. Ophthalmology 1986;93:681–689
38. Grove AS. Wegener's disease. In: Gold DH, Weingeist T, eds. The eye in systemic disease. Philadelphia: Lippincott, 1990:74–76
39. Venning MC, Arfeen S, Bird AG. Antibodies to neutrophil cytoplasmic antigen in systemic vasculitis. Lancet 1987;2:850
40. Bullen CL, Liesegang TJ, McDonald TJ, DeRemee RA. Ocular complications of Wegener's granulomatosis. Ophthalmology 1983;90:279–290
41. Straatsma BR. Ocular manifestations of Wegener's granulomatosis. Am J Ophthalmol 1957;44:789–799
42. Schmidt R, Koderisch J, Krastel H, et al. Sicca syndrome in patients with Wegener's granulomatosis. Lancet 1989;1:904–905
43. Fauci AS. The vasculitis syndromes. In: Wilson JD, Braunwald E, Isselbacher KJ, eds. Harrison's principles of internal medicine. New York: McGraw-Hill, 1991: 1456–1463
44. Waldenström J. Klinisker metoder for pavisanda av hyperproteinami arch deras praktiska varde to diagnostiken. Nord Med 1934;20:2288–2295
45. Ferreiro JE, Pasarin G, Quesada R, Gould E. Benign hypergammaglobulinemic purpura of Waldenström associated with Sjögren's syndrome. Am J Med 1986; 81:734–740
46. Goltz RW, Good RA. Benign hyperglobulinemic purpura. Arch Dermatol 1961; 83:26–38
47. Golding PL, Brown R, Mason AMS, Taylor E. Sicca complex in liver disease. Br Med J 1970;4:340–342
48. Podolsky DK, Isselbacher KJ. Cirrhosis of the liver. In: Wilson JD, Braunwald E, Isselbacher KJ, et al, eds. Harrison's principles of internal medicine. New York: McGraw-Hill, 1991:1340–1350
49. Hansen BU, Lindgren S, Eriksson S, et al. Clinical and immunological features of Sjögren's syndrome in patients with primary biliary cirrhosis with emphasis on focal sialadenitis. Acta Med Scand 1988;224:611–619
50. Franklin RM, Kenyon KR, Tutschka PJ, et al. Ocular manifestations of graft vs. host disease. Ophthalmology 1983;90:4–13
51. Jack MK, Hicks JD. Ocular complications in high dose chemoradiotherapy and marrow transplantation. Ann Ophthalmol 1981;13:709–711
52. Hirst LW, Jabs DA, Tutschka PJ, et al. The eye in bone marrow transplantation. Arch Ophthalmol 1983;101:580–584
53. Gratwhol AA, Moutsopoulos HM, Chused TM, et al. Sjögren-type syndrome after allogenic bone marrow transplantation. Ann Intern Med 1977;87:703–706
54. Lawley TJ, Peck GL, Moutsopoulos HM, et al. Scleroderma, Sjögren-like syndrome, and chronic graft versus host disease. Ann Intern Med 1977;87:707–709
55. Lucca JA, Farris RL, Bielory L, Caputo AR. Keratoconjunctivitis sicca in male

patients infected with human immunodeficiency virus type I. Ophthalmology 1990;97:1008–1010
56. Khadem M, Kalish SB, Goldsmith J, et al. Ophthalmologic findings in acquired immune deficiency syndrome. Arch Ophthalmol 1984;102:201–206
57. Couderc LJ, D'Agay MF, Danon F, et al. Sicca complex and infection with human immunodeficiency virus. Arch Intern Med 1987;147:898–901
58. Mayers M. Ocular sarcoidosis. Int Ophthalmol Clin 1990;30:257–263
59. Crick RP, Hoyle C, Smellie H. The eyes in sarcoidosis. Br J Ophthalmol 1961;45: 461–481
60. Drosos AA, Constantopoulos SH, Psychos D, et al. The forgotten cause of sicca complex; sarcoidosis. J Rheumatol 1989;16:1548–1551
61. Baarsma GS, La Hey E, Glasius E, et al. The predictive value of serum angiotensin converting enzyme and lysozyme levels in the diagnosis of ocular sarcoidosis. Am J Ophthalmol 1987;104:211–217
62. Karma A. Ophthalmologic changes in sarcoidosis. Acta Ophthalmol [Suppl] (Copenh) 1979;141:1–94
63. Vazquez M, Teruel JL. Sicca syndrome due to amyloidosis. J Oral Maxillofac Surg 1988;46:1013–1014
64. Bennett TO, Sugar J, Sahgal S. Ocular manifestations of toxic epidermal necrolysis associated with allopurinol use. Arch Ophthalmol 1977;95:1362–1364
65. Patz A. Ocular involvement in erythema multiforme. Arch Ophthalmol 1950; 43:244–256
66. Ostler HB, Conant MA, Groundwater J. Lyell's disease, the Stevens-Johnson syndrome and exfoliative dermatitis. Trans Am Acad Ophthalmol Otolaryngol 1970; 74:1254–1264
67. Hardy KM, Perry HO, Pingree GC, Kirby TJ. Benign mucous membrane pemphigoid. Arch Dermatol 1971;104:467–475
68. Mondino BJ, Brown SI. Ocular cicatricial pemphigoid. Ophthalmology 1981;88: 95–100
69. Lemp MA, Mahwood MA, Weiler HH. Association of rosacea and keratoconjunctivitis sicca. Arch Ophthalmol 1984;102:556–557
70. Alexander GE, Provost TT, Stevens MB, Alexander EL. Sjögren's syndrome: central nervous system manifestations. Neurology (NY) 1981;31:1391–1396
71. Miro J, Pena-Sagredo JL, Berciano J, et al. Prevalence of primary Sjögren's syndrome in patients with multiple sclerosis. Ann Neurol 1990;27:582–584
72. Noseworthy JH, Bass BH, Vandervoort MK, et al. The prevalence of primary Sjögren's syndrome in a multiple sclerosis population. Ann Neurol 1989;25:95–98
73. Riley CM. Familial dysautonomia. Adv Pediatr 1957;9:157–190
74. Dunnington JH. Congenital alacrima in familial autonomic dysfunction. Arch Ophthalmol 1954;52:925–931
75. Metz HS, Rosenbaum AL. Pediatric ophthalmology. Garden City: Medical Examination Publishing, 1982:193
76. Brunt PW, McKusick VA. Familial dysautonomia: a report of genetic and clinical studies with a review of the literature. Medicine (Baltimore) 1970;49:343
77. Nirankari VS, Khurana RK, Lakhanpal V. Ocular manifestations of Shy-Drager syndrome. Ann Ophthalmol 1982;14:635–638
78. Mausolf FA, ed. The eye and systemic disease. St Louis: Mosby, 1975:314–315
79. Spencer WH, ed. Ophthalmic pathology. Philadelphia: Saunders, 1985:169–170
80. Konig H, Gassman HB, Jenzer G. Ocular involvement in benign botulism B. Am J Ophthalmol 1975;80:430–432
81. Robertson DM, Sizemore GW, Gordon H. Thickened corneal nerves as a manifestation of multiple endocrine neoplasia. Trans Am Acad Ophthalmol Otolaryngol 1975;79:772–787

82. Sommer A, Sugana T. Corneal xerophthalmia and keratomalacia. Arch Ophthalmol 1982;100:404–411
83. Sommer A, Emran N, Tamba T. Vitamin A responsive punctate keratopathy in xerophthalmia. Am J Ophthalmol 1979;87:330–334
84. McLaren DS. Nutritional ophthalmology. New York: Academic, 1980:46–118
85. Keenum DG, Semba RD, Wirasasmita S, et al. Assessment of vitamin A status by a disk applicator for conjunctival impression cytology. Arch Ophthalmol 1990; 108:1436–1441
86. Lawrence DJ, Bern HA. Vitamin A and mucous metaplasia. Ann NY Acad Sci 1963;106:646–653
87. Holly FJ, Lemp MA. Tear physiology and dry eyes. Surv Ophthalmol 1977; 22:69–87
88. Walsh FB, Hoyt WF. Clinical neuro-ophthalmology. Baltimore: Williams & Wilkins, 1969:551–557
89. Gilbard JP, Rossi SR. Tear film and ocular surface changes in a rabbit model of neurotrophic keratitis. Ophthalmology 1990;97:308–312
90. Gancher S. Parkinson's disease. In: Fraunfelder FT, Roy FH, eds. Current ocular therapy. Philadelphia: Saunders, 1990:263–264
91. Fraunfelder FT, ed. Drug-induced ocular side effects and drug interactions. Philadelphia: Lea & Febiger, 1989:513–514
92. Lemp MA. Tear film: new concept and implications for the management of the dry eye. Transactions of the New Orleans Academy of Ophthalmology. New York: Raven, 1987:53–64

Systemic Associations of Corneal Deposits

Robert C. Arffa, M.D.
F. Rodney Eve, M.D., F.R.C.S.

A wide variety of systemic diseases can be associated with corneal deposits (Table 1). In many cases, the deposits are the first indication of the presence of the disease or are an important accessible part of the diagnosis. For instance, the most frequent clinical sign in Fabry's disease is corneal epithelial deposits, which are asymptomatic but clearly visible at the slit-lamp biomicroscope. Likewise, the presence of a Kayser-Fleischer ring is important in differentiating between patients with Wilson's disease and those with other neurological and hepatic diseases. Conjunctival or corneal biopsy is a relatively accessible means of diagnosing many inborn errors of metabolism once the ophthalmologist is alerted to the possibility of the disease by its characteristic corneal findings [1].

Deposition of materials in the cornea can occur for a variety of reasons. Excess serum levels can lead to deposition in many body tissues and, due to its transparency, the cornea is often the tissue in which the deposits are most evident. Specific binding to corneal structures can facilitate accumulation. Many of the systemic diseases associated with corneal deposits are inborn disorders of metabolism. In most of these, an enzyme is either absent or deficient. If an enzyme normally active in corneal cells is deficient, its substrate accumulates, causing opacification.

Superficial corneal opacification also occurs in many skin diseases [1]. Since these are not true deposits, they are listed in Table 1 but are not discussed in the text. The corneal layers most typically containing deposits in each systemic disease are listed in Table 2.

To understand the pathogenesis of these deposits, it is useful to classify the diseases according to the source of the deposits, whether the deposited material comes from elsewhere in the body (exogenous) or is produced within the cornea (endogenous), and the chemical nature of the deposits (Table 3).

Exogenous Deposits

Deposits of exogenous substances most often occur because of excess serum levels. In many cases, this is due to enzyme deficiency, but drug or mineral

Table 1 *Systemic Associations of Corneal Deposits*

Corneal dystrophies
Lattice corneal dystrophy type II (Meretoja's syndrome)
Macular dystrophy
Central stromal crystalline dystrophy (Schnyder's dystrophy)
Immunological disorders
Multiple myeloma and other dysproteinemias
Langerhans cell granulomatosis
Metabolic disorders
Hypercalcemia
Lipid metabolism
Sphingolipidoses
Hyperlipoproteinemia
Tangier disease
Farber's disease
Apoprotein A-1 deficiency
Lecithin cholesterol acyltransferase deficiency
Fish-eye disease
Carbohydrate metabolism
Mucopolysaccharidoses
Von Gierke disease
Combined carbohydrate and lipid metabolism
Mucolipidoses
Glycoprotein storage disorders
Disorders of amino acid metabolism
Cystinosis
Tyrosinemia II (Richner-Hanhart syndrome)
Others
Amyloidosis
Wilson's disease
Hyperuricemia
Zellweger syndrome
Systemic medications
Gold
Phenothiazines
Aminoquinolones
Quinacrine
Thioxanthenes
Amiodarone
Miscellaneous other agents
Skin diseases
Ichthyosis
Kyrle's disease
Keratosis follicularis (Darier's disease)
Acrodermatitis enteropathica
Melkersson-Rosenthal syndrome
Cutis verticis gyrata (Rosenthal-Kloepfer syndrome)
Dermochondrocorneal dystrophy of François
Epidermal nevus syndrome
Pili torti
Anhidrotic ectodermal dysplasia

administration, malignancy, dietary excess, and many other abnormalities may be responsible. Deposition usually occurs in many body tissues, but the cornea is the tissue in which the deposits are most readily visible. Specific corneal deposition can be caused by the increased light exposure, hypertonicity, and increased pH of tears, and the lack of blood vessels. In the diseased state, the presence of abnormal, leaky vessels, inflammation, and reparative processes can promote deposition.

Exogenous substances can enter the cornea by three routes: limbal vessels, aqueous humor, or tears. Influx from limbal vessels leads mainly to stromal accumulation, greater in the peripheral than in the central cornea. Similarly, substances in the aqueous enter mainly the posterior layers, and substances in the tears affect the epithelium primarily.

Lipid

Lipid is certainly the most common exogenous material deposited in the cornea. In the form of corneal arcus (arcus senilis), it usually is not associated with systemic disease, but it can be associated with hyperlipoproteinemia. Lipid degeneration occurs primarily in the presence of abnormal corneal vessels, but hyperlipoproteinemia plays a role in some patients. Also, several rare disorders of lipid metabolism can be associated with corneal lipid deposition.

Arcus Arcus consists of extracellular deposits of cholesterol, cholesterol esters, phospholipids, and triglycerides in the peripheral corneal stroma. It is a phenomenon associated with aging, seen in 60% of people 60 years of age, and in more than 90% of those older than 80 [2]. The formation of the lipid deposits is related to increasing age, proximity of blood vessels to the peripheral cornea, a high degree of vessel permeability, and elevation of serum cholesterol and low-density lipoproteins (LDLs) [3–8]. The permeability of the limbal vessels probably increases with age, and low-density lipids pass more readily into the peripheral cornea. This process is accentuated in the presence of high serum levels or abnormally increased permeability.

Corneal arcus generally is not indicative of systemic disease, though some cases are related to hyperlipoproteinemia, particularly types II and III [4]. The presence of arcus in someone younger than 50 years is a significant risk factor for coronary heart disease [9]. Premature arcus formation also occurs in lethicin cholesterol acyltransferase (LCAT) deficiency and phytosterolemia [10].

LCAT Deficiency LCAT deficiency is a rare autosomally inherited deficiency of plasma LCAT, an enzyme that normally esterifies cholesterol. A reduction in its activity results in elevations of serum unesterified cholesterol, very low density lipoprotein (VLDL), triglycerides, and phospholipids. The structures of all lipoproteins are abnormal.

Beginning in early childhood, corneal opacities consisting of many small gray dots can be seen throughout the stroma. There is a lucid interval at the limbus, and the opacities can become dense in the periphery, resembling a corneal arcus [11–16]. Occasionally, crystals—presumably cholesterol—can be seen at the edges of the deposits. Visual acuity is not affected. Histopatho-

Table 2 *Level of Corneal Deposits*

Condition	Epithelium	Bowman's Layer	Stroma	Descemet's Membrane	Endothelium
Corneal dystrophies					
Lattice corneal dystrophy type II			X		
Macular dystrophy			X		X
Central stromal crystalline dystrophy			X		
Immunological disorders					
Multiple myeloma	X		X		
Langerhans cell granulomatosis			X		
Metabolic disorders					
Hypercalcemia	X	X			
Sphingolipidoses	X	X[a]	X[a]		X[a]
Hyperlipoproteinemia			X		
Tangier disease			X		
Farber's disease	X		X		
Apoprotein A-1 deficiency			X		
Lecithin cholesterol acyltransferase deficiency			X		
Fish-eye disease			X		
Mucopolysaccharidoses	X[a]		X		X
Mucolipidoses	X		X		
Glycoprotein storage disorders	X		X		

Cystinosis	X		X	
Tyrosinemia II	X			
Wilson's disease				X
Hyperuricemia	X	X		
Systemic medications				
Gold	X	X		
Phenothiazines	X			X
Aminoquinolones	X			
Amiodarone	X			
Skin diseases				
Ichthyosis			X	X
Kyrle's disease	X[b]			
Keratosis follicularis (Darier's disease)	X		X	
Acrodermatitis enteropathica	X[b]	X		
Melkersson-Rosenthal syndrome	X	X		
Dermochondrocorneal dystrophy of François	X[b]			
Epidermal nevus syndrome				
Pili torti				
Anhidrotic ectodermal dysplasia	X			

[a]Deposits evident only on microscopy.
[b]Subepithelial.

Table 3 *Types of Deposits*

Exogenous deposits
Lipid
Hyperlipoproteinemia
?Central stromal crystalline dystrophy (Schnyder's dystrophy)
?Tangier disease
?Apoprotein A-1 deficiency
?Lecithin cholesterol acyltransferase deficiency
?Fish-eye disease
Protein
Multiple myeloma and other dysproteinemias
Hyperuricemia
Minerals
Hypercalcemia
Wilson's disease
Gold therapy
Drugs
Phenothiazines
Aminoquinolones
Quinacrine
Amiodarone
Indomethacin
Clofazimine
Tamoxifen
Many others
Endogenous deposits
Protein
Cystinosis
Tyrosinemia
?Lattice corneal dystrophy
Lipid
Sphingolipidoses
Farber's disease
Carbohydrate
Glycogen storage diseases
Carbohydrate and protein
Mucopolysaccharidoses
Macular dystrophy
Glycoprotein storage diseases
Combined carbohydrate, lipid, and protein
Mucolipidoses
Glycoprotein storage disorders

logical examination shows vacuoles containing membranous deposits within keratocytes.

Tangier Disease Tangier disease, or familial high-density lipoprotein (HDL) deficiency, is another rare autosomal recessive disorder of lipid metabolism [17]. There is an absence or reduction of plasma alpha-HDL; an abnormal HDL is found instead. Cholesterol esters accumulate in many tissues, particularly in reticuloendothelial cells. A yellowish orange tinge of the tonsils, rectal mucosa, and conjunctiva can be seen.

There is diffuse stromal clouding of the cornea caused by the intracellular deposition of cholesterol esters [13, 18]. It appears as many small dots throughout the stroma, sometimes in a whorllike pattern, densest posteriorly and in the horizontal meridian. A distinct arcus is not present, and the vision is not affected.

Fish-Eye Disease Fish-eye disease is a rare inherited disorder in which marked corneal clouding is the most prominent finding. The exact biochemical defect is not known, but HDL levels are low (10% of normal), and LDL, triglyceride, and VLDL levels are elevated [19, 20]. The eyes are said to resemble those of boiled fish. Beginning late in the second decade, gray-white-yellow dots are seen throughout the stroma, densest in the periphery. They can become sufficiently dense as to require keratoplasty. On histopathological examination, numerous extracellular vacuoles of cholesterol-containing lipid are seen throughout the stroma [20].

Central Stromal Crystalline Dystrophy (of Schnyder) Central stromal crystalline dystrophy is an autosomal dominant corneal dystrophy in which there is progressive deposition of cholesterol and neutral fats in the central cornea. Fine needle-shaped polychromatic crystals are seen in the central anterior corneal stroma, in a round, oval, discoid, or annular configuration (Fig 1) [1, 21–25]. A dense arcus and limbal girdle of Vogt occur in many cases [26].

Hyperlipidemia is present in a significant portion of the patients, but the type and severity of the hyperlipidemia varies [22, 24], even within families, and there is no relation between serum lipoprotein levels and progression of the disease [27]. Chondrodystrophy and genu valgum are also present in some families [22, 24, 26, 28].

This disease is most likely a localized disorder of cholesterol metabolism, and it may be exacerbated by systemic hyperlipoproteinemia.

Other Disorders Apoprotein A-1 deficiency is an extremely rare disorder of lipid metabolism in which diffuse corneal clouding occurs [29]. Corneal opacities are also seen in Farber's disease (see page 103), another inborn error of lipid metabolism.

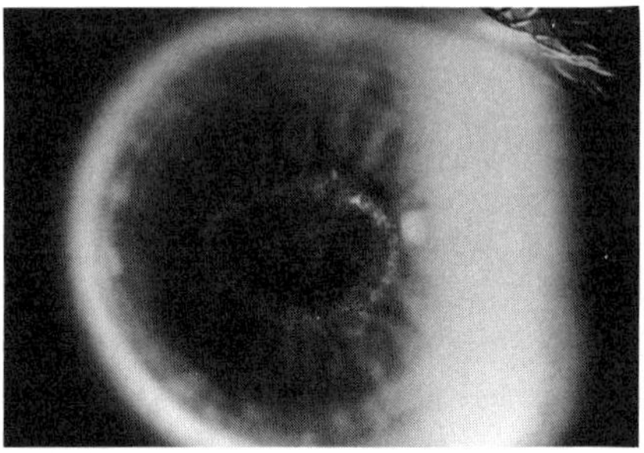

Figure 1 *Corneal deposits in Schnyder's central stromal crystalline dystrophy.*

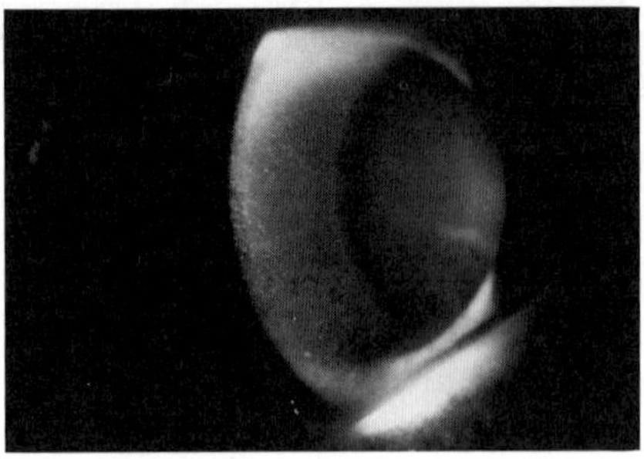

Figure 2 *Crystalline and sheetlike epithelial deposits in multiple myeloma.*

Protein

Multiple Myeloma and the Dysproteinemias Multiple myeloma is a neoplastic proliferation of plasma cells that most commonly becomes manifest between 40 and 70 years of age [30, 31]. Systemic findings include multiple osteolytic lesions, susceptibility to bacterial infections, anemia, pathological fractures, hypercalcemia, renal failure, and hyperviscosity. The abnormal plasma cells produce immunoglobulins, and their components, particularly light chains, can become deposited in tissues.

Crystals can be seen in the conjunctiva, cornea, and retina [32]. In the cornea, they appear as fine punctate or needlelike, multicolored crystals in the corneal epithelium or anterior stroma (Fig 2) [32, 33]. In some cases, a diffuse stromal haze is present. In other cases, amorphous gray-white epithelial and subepithelial deposits are seen in the corneal periphery, usually superiorly [34–36]. Similar changes can be seen in patients with other forms of dysproteinemia, such as benign monoclonal gammopathy [37–39], and essential cryoglobulinemia [35].

In most cases, vision is only mildly reduced. Histologically, corneal crystals composed of immunoglobulin-related proteins have been found in keratocytes and epithelium [37, 38, 40].

Band keratopathy can be seen in association with hypercalcemia, and a polychromatic, dustlike deposition of copper centrally in Descemet's membrane can be seen. The latter appears to be related to the ability of some myeloma proteins to bind copper [41].

Alkaptonuria Alkaptonuria is a rare hereditary disorder of metabolism due to the absence of the enzyme homogentisic acid oxidase, which is involved in the catabolism of tyrosine and phenylalanine. Its absence results in the accumulation of homogentisic acid, which can become oxidized to form pigmented polymers (alkapton), and the acid and the polymers can bind collagen. The resulting yellow-brown pigmentation of cartilaginous tissues is called *ochronosis.*

One of the earliest manifestations is scleral pigmentation, which usually is seen in the interpalpebral zone beginning in the third to fifth decades of life [42–46]. The conjunctiva, episclera, tendons of the horizontal recti and, less commonly, peripheral cornea can also become pigmented. The corneal deposits are located in the deep epithelium, Bowman's layer, and anterior stroma. The pigment is usually brownish black, and the deposits look like oil droplets, similar to those seen in spheroidal degeneration.

Amyloidosis Amyloid is an extracellular proteinaceous hyaline material that can be deposited in various tissues in the body as part of a localized or systemic disease. Corneal deposits most commonly are degenerative, secondary to localized disease, usually either trauma or chronic inflammation. *Lattice corneal dystrophy* is a term used for a group of hereditary forms of amyloidosis. In most forms of lattice dystrophy, the amyloid deposits are limited to the cornea; however, in one type (known as *type II lattice dystrophy, Meretoja's syndrome,* or *familial amyloid polyneuropathy type IV*), involvement of the skin and cranial and peripheral nerves is seen [47–50]. The latticelike corneal changes usually become manifest between 20 and 35 years of age, and they tend to be milder than in the more common lattice type I. Fewer lattice lines (eight to twenty) are present, good vision is retained until the seventh decade, and erosive symptoms are less frequent.

Histologically, a thin layer of amyloid deposits is seen posterior to Bowman's layer, and linear deposits of amyloid appear to have replaced corneal nerves [48]. The amyloid protein has not been identified but is related to transthyretin [51].

Minerals

Calcium Calcium deposition in the cornea most commonly accompanies localized ocular disease, particularly chronic intraocular inflammation; however, it can also occur in hypercalcemia. Hypercalcemia is seen in a wide variety of systemic disorders that cause increased calcium absorption from the gut, increased resorption of bone, or decreased calcium excretion by the kidneys.

The exact mechanism of calcium deposition in the cornea has not been determined, but some factors have been identified [1, 52, 53]. In many tissues, calcium and phosphate concentrations are very close to those that favor precipitation. Mild elevation of either calcium or phosphate levels, or an increase in pH, can lead to precipitation. Evaporation of tears may favor calcium precipitation by increasing the local ion concentration and by making the pH more alkaline. Carbon dioxide is lost from the tears in the palpebral fissure, and this may locally elevate pH. The lack of blood vessels in the cornea may also prevent the normal buffering ability of blood serum to inhibit variations in tissue pH [52]. Intraocular inflammation can promote this process by altering corneal metabolism, resulting in a rise in tissue pH and thus favoring precipitation of calcium salts [54, 55].

Clinically, calcium deposition is seen as band keratopathy, grayish white superficial deposits in the interpalpebral cornea. It usually begins in the periphery and gradually extends centrally. A lucid interval is seen between the calcific band and the limbus. Small holes are present within the opacity, giving it a Swiss-cheese appearance.

Treatment includes return of serum calcium levels to normal, control of intraocular inflammation, and removal of calcium deposits by EDTA chelation.

Copper Corneal copper deposition occurs in Wilson's disease and other liver diseases. Wilson's disease is an inherited disorder in which copper excretion into bile is impaired, with accumulation of copper in the liver and eventual spillover into the blood and deposition in other tissues. The exact metabolic defect is not known. Most manifestations are related to liver dysfunction or neurological impairment, due to copper deposition. The major site of neural deposition is the basal ganglia.

In Wilson's disease, copper deposition can be seen in the cornea as the Kayser-Fleischer ring and in the lens as "sunflower cataracts." The Kayser-Fleischer ring is a yellow-brown, green, or red peripheral band, 1 to 3 mm wide, at the level of Descemet's membrane (Fig 3) [56–58]. The deposition is first noted superiorly, in the most peripheral portion of Descemet's. Gonioscopic examination is sometimes required to detect it.

A Kayser-Fleischer ring is seen in approximately 95% of patients with Wilson's disease [59–61]. It also can be seen in some patients with primary biliary cirrhosis, progressive intrahepatic cholestasis of childhood, chronic active hepatitis with cirrhosis, other cholestatic syndromes, and exogenous chalcosis [62–64]. Patients with Wilson's disease can be differentiated from those with these other disorders by their inability to incorporate radioactive copper into ceruloplasmin [59].

Gold Gold can accumulate in the cornea and conjunctiva after prolonged administration in the treatment of rheumatoid arthritis and other collagen vascular diseases [65–69]. The presence of deposits is related to the total dose of gold, the duration of treatment, and the intensity of therapy (total dose divided by duration of therapy) [67]. Deposition is usually seen with total doses in excess of 1 gm. The deposits usually clear within 3 to 6 months after cessation of treatment, suggesting a dynamic process of deposition and removal [65].

Both corneal stromal and epithelial deposition can occur. Stromal deposits are seen as fine, dustlike, yellow or purple-violet granules that are more numerous in the deeper layers and inferiorly. Epithelial deposits are usually diffuse, sometimes with a vortex pattern, but may also be peripheral or only central [68]. Marginal infiltrative or ulcerative keratitis can also occur, possibly as a hypersensitivity reaction to the gold [1, 70].

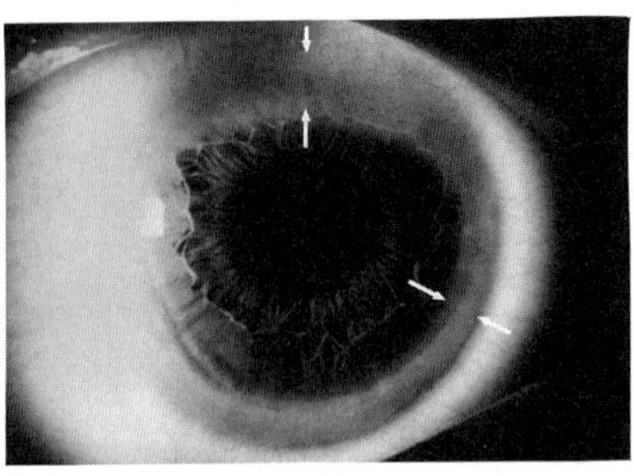

Figure 3 *Kayser-Fleischer ring* (arrows) *in Wilson's disease.*

Uric Acid

Hyperuricemia occurs in a wide variety of disorders. The term *gout* is used for the combination of hyperuricemia and any of the following: characteristic arthritis, urate deposition in joints (tophi), interstitial renal disease, or uric acid nephrolithiasis. This also occurs in a heterogeneous group of disorders, often caused by a combination of genetic and environmental influences. In hyperuricemia of any cause, urate crystals can become deposited in cartilage, epiphyseal bone, tendons, synovial membranes, kidneys, and other tissues. Uric acid deposition in the cornea may be promoted by alkaline pH, decreased temperature, and concentration by evaporation, mechanisms similar to those that can promote calcium deposition.

In the eye, deposition can affect the cornea, conjunctiva, sclera, and tarsal plates of the lids [71–74]. Monosodium urate crystals can be deposited in the corneal epithelium and superficial stroma. They are fine, punctate or needle-like, and refractile, and are most dense in the palpebral fissure [75]. The appearance can be similar to that of band keratopathy, but the deposits are brownish rather than whitish gray. Histologically, the urate crystals are found in the nuclei of epithelial cells and in the superficial stroma [75]. The corneal deposits can be removed by scraping or superficial keratectomy [71].

Acute conjunctival inflammation, scleritis, episcleritis, and iritis can also be seen [73]. These episodes may be associated with acute attacks of gouty arthritis but, overall, are extremely rare in patients with gout.

Drugs

Drug-Related Vortex Keratopathy Chronic systemic administration of certain drugs can lead to deposits in the corneal epithelium that can be seen with the slit-lamp biomicroscope (Table 4). These typically produce a vortex or verticillate pattern (Fig 4). The deposits range in color from gray to yellow-brown and rarely interfere with vision. They are dose-related and reversible after cessation of the drug.

Many of the drugs associated with this picture exhibit cationic amphophilia, and it has been hypothesized that these drugs form complexes with polar intracellular lipids, which then cannot be metabolized by lysosomal phospholipases [76, 77]. The complexes accumulate in the epithelial cells, resulting in an appearance similar to that of Fabry's disease.

Other Drugs and Stromal Deposits Many other drugs can be associated with stromal deposits [1]. A partial listing is given in Table 4. Usually, they give rise to finely granular deposits within the corneal stroma. The deposits are dose-related and reversible.

■ Endogenous Deposits

Substances abnormally accumulate in the cornea in many inborn systemic disorders of metabolism. The biochemical lesion, in most cases in which the

Table 4 *Drugs Associated with Corneal Deposits*

Epithelial deposits	*Stromal deposits*
Aminoquinolones	Antacids
Amodiaquine	Gold
Chloroquine	Indomethacin
Hydroxychloroquine	Phenothiazines
Clofazimine	Phenylbutazone
Indomethacin	Practolol
Naproxen	Retinoids
Perhexiline	Silver
Suramin	
Tamoxifen	
Thioxanthines	
Chlorprothixine	
Thiothixine	
Tilorone	

defect has been identified, is an abnormal or deficient enzyme. Manifestations are caused by the accumulation of the normal substrate of this enzyme and the deficiency of the normal product. Most of the enzyme deficiencies that have been elucidated affect enzymes involved in catabolism. One class of catabolic disorders that commonly affects the cornea is the lysosomal storage disorders, in which the abnormal enzyme is an acid hydrolase found within lysosomes. The substrate of the abnormal enzyme, usually a complex lipid or polysaccharide, accumulates in swollen lysosomes in specific tissues.

Corneal accumulation of endogenous products occurs if the enzyme is normally active in corneal cells (epithelium, keratocytes, or endothelium) and the enzyme substrate is normally present in the cornea. The most common corneal manifestation in metabolic disease is loss of clarity due to accumulation of the metabolic products. However, the excess material can also cause cellular injury and lead to epithelial erosions or vascularization.

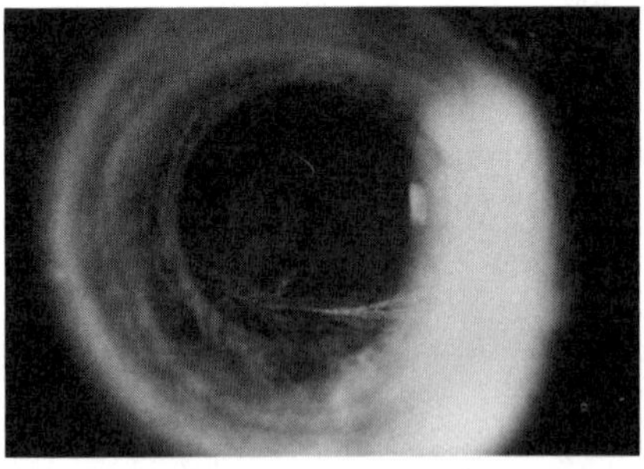

Figure 4 *Verticillate corneal epithelial deposits with amiodarone administration.*

Most hereditary corneal dystrophies are probably enzyme deficiencies, in which the only manifestation is ocular. For example, macular corneal deficiency results from impaired synthesis of keratan sulfate, with accumulation of precursors producing corneal opacification [78–81]. There are no extraocular manifestations of the disease, but keratan sulfate is also absent from serum and cartilage [82, 83].

Disorders of Amino Acid Metabolism

Cystinosis Cystinosis is a rare autosomal recessive inherited disorder characterized by the accumulation of cystine in tissues throughout the body. It occurs in infantile, juvenile, and adult forms, with decreasing severity, respectively. The transport of cystine out of lysosomes is impaired, resulting in the formation of intracellular (intralysosomal) cystine crystals. These crystals are most readily observed in the cornea, because of its transparency. They form in both the corneal epithelium and keratocytes.

Corneal involvement is evidenced by glistening, polychromatic, needlelike to rectangular crystals in the stroma (Fig 5). They tend to be more pronounced anteriorly than posteriorly and more numerous peripherally than centrally [84]. In the infantile form, they first appear from 6 to 15 months of age. In the adult form, they may become evident in the teen years or not until 50 years. In each form, they continually become denser with age [85, 86].

The crystals are associated with photophobia but do not decrease acuity. In advanced cases, corneal erosions can occur and the cornea can become thickened [87].

Topically administered cysteamine (beta-mercaptoethylamine) can reduce corneal crystal content. The cysteamine reacts with intracellular cystine, forming a cysteine-cysteamine disulfide that resembles lysine and is transported out of the lysosome by the normal lysine transport system. The cysteamine is given as a 10 mM drop hourly during the day [88–90].

Tyrosinemia II Tyrosinemia II (Richner-Hanhart syndrome) is an autosomal recessive disorder of tyrosine metabolism that appears to be due to a

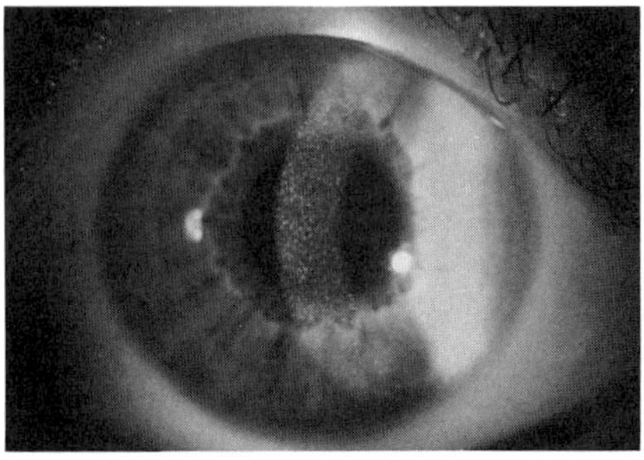

Figure 5 *Corneal crystals in cystinosis.*

deficiency of tyrosine aminotransferase [91]. In most cells, the excess tyrosine is removed by mitochondrial aspartate transaminase, but this enzyme is not present in cells of ectodermal origin. Accumulation of tyrosine in ectodermal cells results in hyperkeratosis, blisters, and erosions, most noted on the palms, soles, knees, elbows, and corneas [92]. Institution of a diet low in tyrosine and phenylalanine can lead to resolution of the eye and skin lesions.

Corneal intraepithelial and subepithelial opacifications occur, sometimes with erosions or ulcerations [91–96]. Thick plaques can form and can take on a dendritic or sunburst appearance [97]. Photophobia, tearing, redness, and pain are often present.

In experimental models, tyrosine crystals are found in the affected epithelium [98]. Theoretically, the crystals form in lysosomes and result in their destabilization. Proteolytic enzymes are released, causing cellular injury and stimulating inflammatory cell infiltration and vascularization [99]. Why tyrosine crystals stimulate inflammation but not cystine crystals is unclear.

Disorders of Lysosomal Enzymes

Mucopolysaccharidoses Mucopolysaccharides, also called *glycosaminoglycans,* are components of the extracellular matrix in many tissues, including the cornea. They are complexes of carbohydrate and protein in which the polysaccharide component is more prominent than the protein. The major acid mucopolysaccharides in the corneal stroma are keratan sulfate, chondroitin, chondroitin sulfate, and dermatan sulfate. The mucopolysaccharidoses are recessively inherited deficiencies of lysosomal enzymes that hydrolyze mucopolysaccharides [100–105]. Deficiencies in enzymes that normally degrade dermatan sulfate or keratan sulfate lead to accumulation of these substances in the cornea, resulting in corneal clouding.

Hurler's syndrome is the classic form in which there is a deficiency of alpha-L-iduronidase, resulting in accumulation of heparan sulfate and dermatan sulfate. It is characterized by gargoylelike facies, marked skeletal abnormalities (dysostosis multiplex), and progressive mental retardation. Beginning in infancy, fine, gray punctate opacities are seen in the anterior stroma first and then in the posterior stroma and endothelium, resulting in a diffuse, ground-glass haze (Fig 6). Corneal thickness may be increased.

Corneal opacification is also seen in types IS (Scheie), IH/S (Hurler-Scheie compound), II (Hunter), IV (Morquio), VI (Maroteaux-Lamy), and VII (Sly).

Mucolipidoses Mucolipidoses are lysosomal storage diseases involving some combination of mucopolysaccharide, glycoprotein, glycolipid, and oligosaccharide metabolism. Mucolipidosis types II (I cell disease) and III are due to a defect in the posttranslational processing of lysosomal enzymes. The abnormal enzyme (UDP-*N*-acetylglucosamine (GLcNAc):glycoprotein GLcNAc 1-phosphotransferase) is involved in the posttranslational synthesis of a recognition marker, which normally binds the enzyme to a receptor in the lysosome. In the absence of this marker, the lysosomal enzymes are secreted into the extracellular space instead of binding to the lysosome [106]. All cells in the body are deficient in activity of the phototransferase, but only cells of mesen-

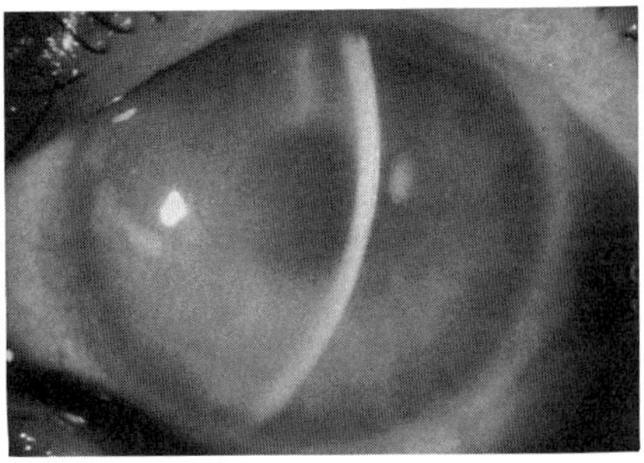

Figure 6 *Diffuse corneal clouding in mucopolysaccharidosis.*

chymal origin (e.g., fibroblasts) are deficient in lysosomal enzymes. Therefore, in other cells, alternate methods of transportation of the lysosomal enzymes must be present.

Mucolipidosis types II and III are characterized by gargoylelike facies, growth and psychomotor retardation, thickened skin, and mucopolysaccharidosislike skeletal dysplasia (dysostosis multiplex) [107, 108]. Progressive opacification of the corneal stroma is seen in both types, although it is milder in type III [109–112]. In conjunctival biopsies, striking inclusions can be seen in fibroblasts [110, 113, 114].

Fabry's Disease Fabry's disease is a disorder of glycosphingolipid catabolism. Glycosphingolipids are widely distributed in human tissues as normal surface components of plasma membranes and some intracellular membranes. Those with terminal galactosyl moieties accumulate in Fabry's disease, due to deficiency of ceramide trihexosidase (an alpha-galactosidase) [115, 116]. Endogenous metabolism of membrane material is the major source of accumulated substrate in avascular sites, such as the cornea.

Clinically, Fabry's disease is characterized by telangiectatic skin lesions, hypohidrosis, febrile episodes, peripheral neuropathy, renal failure, cardiovascular disease, gastrointestinal symptoms, and central nervous system disturbances. Corneal epithelial opacification is present in nearly all affected men as well as in 90% of female carriers [117–121]. It is seen as fine, superficial, white, yellow, or brown dots distributed in a vortex pattern. The opacities can be seen only with the aid of a slit-lamp biomicroscope and do not affect vision.

Histologically, intracytoplasmic lamellar inclusions are noted in corneal epithelial cells, stromal keratocytes, Bowman's layer, endothelium, and conjunctival epithelium [121–125].

Farber's Lipogranulomatosis Farber's lipogranulomatosis is due to an inborn deficiency of lysosomal ceramidase. Ceramides are types of sphingolipid that are known to be important in neural tissue and skin and most likely are also present in synovial membranes. Due to a deficiency of lysosomal ceramidase, ceramides accumulate intracellularly and eventually spill over into the extracellular tissue. This material stimulates a granulomatous reaction [126], producing the clinical manifestations.

The manifestations include painful and progressively deformed joints, subcutaneous nodules, hoarseness, nervous system dysfunction, lung, heart, and lymph node involvement, and usually death within a few years. Corneal opacities occur [127], and granulomatous, xanthomalike, conjunctival lesions can be seen in type I [128]. Histologically, granulomas and accumulation of lipid-laden macrophages are noted in affected tissues. Round inclusions, surrounded by a bilaminar membrane, are seen in conjunctival and corneal epithelium and in keratocytes [129].

Glycoprotein Storage Disorders Glycoprotein storage disorders are rare autosomal recessive disorders involving enzymes that hydrolyze polysaccharide linkages. There is a large amount of glycoprotein in normal tissues, including nervous tissue. Therefore, normal turnover produces a large amount of polysaccharide that must be degraded in lysosomes. Oligosaccharides accumulate in mannosidosis and sialidosis; glycolipids, glycopeptides, and oligosaccharides accumulate in fucosidosis. On histopathological examination, membrane-bound inclusions are found in corneal and conjunctival epithelial cells and keratocytes [130–132]. All are characterized by mental retardation, coarse facies, and skeletal dysplasia.

Progressive stromal and epithelial corneal clouding occurs in some patients with sialidosis [133], including those with Goldberg-Cotlier syndrome [130, 134]. Superficial corneal opacities have been reported in a few cases of mannosidosis. Spokelike posterior cortical cataracts are commonly seen [135]. In fucosidosis, dilated, tortuous conjunctival vessels and central anterior corneal opacification have been reported [136, 137].

Disorders of Carbohydrate Metabolism

Glycogen storage disease type 1A (von Gierke disease) is an autosomal recessive disorder in which the enzyme glucose-6-phosphatase is deficient. This enzyme is important in the conversion of glycogen to glucose and, in its absence, glucose deficiency and glycogen accumulation in tissues is seen. It is marked by hypoglycemia, hepatomegaly, bleeding diathesis, hyperlipidemia, and short stature. A faint brown peripheral corneal clouding may be present.

■ References

1. Arffa RC. Grayson's diseases of the cornea. St Louis: Mosby, 1991
2. Duke-Elder S, Leigh AG. Diseases of the outer eye: vol 8, system of ophthalmology. St Louis: Mosby, 1965:873
3. Walton KW. Studies on the pathogenesis of corneal arcus formation. J Pathol 1973;111:263–274
4. Vinger PF, Sachs BA. Ocular manifestations of hyperlipoproteinaemia. Am J Ophthalmol 1970;70:563–573
5. Rifkind BM. Corneal arcus and hyperlipoproteinaemia. Surv Ophthalmol 1972; 16:295–304
6. Walton KW, Dunkerley DJ. Studies on the pathogenesis of corneal arcus formation: II. Immunofluorescent studies on lipid deposition in the eye of the lipid-fed rabbit. J Pathol 1974;114:217–229

7. Winder AF. Factors influencing the variable expression of xanthelasmata and corneal arcus in familial hypercholesterolemia. Birth Defects 1982;18:449–462
8. Pe'er J, Vidaurri J, Halfon ST, et al. Association between corneal arcus and some of the risk factors for coronary artery disease. Br J Ophthalmol 1983;67:795–798
9. Rosenman RH, Brand RJ, Sholtz BJ, Jenkins CD. Relation of corneal arcus to cardiovascular risk factors and incidence of coronary disease. N Engl J Med 1974;291:1322–1324
10. Björkhem I, Skrede S. Familial diseases with storage of sterols other than cholesterol: cerebrotendinous xanthomatosis and phytosterolemia. In: Scriver CR et al, eds. The metabolic basis of inherited disease, ed 6. New York: McGraw-Hill, 1989
11. Gjone E, Bergaust B. Corneal opacity in familial plasma cholesterol ester deficiency. Acta Ophthalmol (Copenh) 1969;47:222–227
12. Horven I, Effe K, Gjone E. Corneal and fundus changes in familial LCAT deficiency. Acta Ophthalmol (Copenh) 1974;52:201–210
13. Bron AJ. Corneal changes in the dyslipoproteinemias. Cornea 1989;8:135–140
14. Bron AJ, Lloyd JK, Fosbrooke AS, et al. Primary LCAT deficiency disease. Lancet 1975;1:928–929
15. Bethell W, McCullocoh C, Ghosh M. Lethicin cholesterol acyltransferase deficiency: light and electron microscopic finding from 2 corneas. Can J Ophthalmol 1975;10:494–501
16. Vrabec MP, Shapiro MB, Koller E, et al. Ophthalmic observations in lecithin cholesterol acyltransferase deficiency. Arch Ophthalmol 1988;106:225–229
17. Hoffman H II, Fredrickson DS. Tangier disease (familial high density lipoprotein deficiency): clinical and genetic features in two adults. Am J Med 1965;39:582–593
18. Chu FC, Kuwabara T, Cogan DG, et al. Ocular manifestations of familial high-density lipoprotein deficiency (Tangier disease). Arch Ophthalmol 1979;97:1926–1928
19. Carlson LA, Phillipson B. Fish-eye disease. Lancet 1979;2:921–923
20. Philipson BT. Fish eye disease. Birth Defects 1982;18:441–448
21. Ehlers N, Matthiessen M. Hereditary crystalline dystrophy of Schnyder. Acta Ophthalmol (Copenh) 1973;51:316–324
22. Luxenburg M. Hereditary crystalline dystrophy of the cornea. Am J Ophthalmol 1967;63:507–511
23. Kaseras A, Price A. Central crystalline corneal dystrophy. Br J Ophthalmol 1970;54:659–662
24. Bron AJ, Williams HP, Carruthers ME. Hereditary crystalline stromal dystrophy of Schnyder: clinical features of a family with hyperlipoproteinemia. Br J Ophthalmol 1972;56:383–399
25. Grop K. Clinical and histologic findings in crystalline corneal dystrophy. Acta Ophthalmol (Copenh) 1973;51(suppl 120):52–57
26. Delleman JW, Winkelman JE. Degeneratio corneae cristallinea hereditaria: a clinical, genetical and histological study. Ophthalmologica 1968;155:409–426
27. Lisch W, Weidle EG, Lisch C, et al. Schnyder's dystrophy: progression and metabolism. Ophthalmic Paediatr Genet 1986;7:45–56
28. Fry WE, Pickett WE. Crystalline dystrophy of the cornea. Trans Am Ophthalmol Soc 1950;48:220–227
29. Breslow JL. Familial disorders of high density lipoprotein metabolism. In: Scriver CR et al, eds. The metabolic basis of inherited disease, ed 6. New York: McGraw-Hill, 1989
30. Azar HA, Potter M. Multiple myeloma and related diseases. Hagerstown, MD: Harper & Row, 1973:1–52
31. Kyle RA. Multiple myeloma: review of 899 cases. Mayo Clin Proc 1975;50:29–40
32. Pinkerton RMH, Robertson DM. Corneal and conjunctival changes in dysproteinemia. Invest Ophthalmol 1969;8:357–364

33. Aronson SB, Shaw R. Corneal crystals in multiple myeloma. Arch Ophthalmol 1959;61:541–546
34. Beebe WE, Webster RG, Spencer WB. Atypical corneal manifestations of multiple myeloma: a clinical histopathologic, and immunohistochemical report. Cornea 1989;8:274–280
35. Kremer I, Wright P, Merin S, et al. Corneal subepithelial monoclonal kappa IgG deposits in essential cryoglobulinaemia. Br J Ophthalmol 1989;73:669–673
36. Hill JC, Mulligan GP. Subepithelial corneal deposits in IgG lambda myeloma. Br J Ophthalmol 1989;73:552–554
37. Rodrigues MM, Krachmer JH, Miller SD, et al. Posterior corneal crystalline deposits in benign monoclonal gammopathy: a clinicopathologic case report. Arch Ophthalmol 1979;97:124–128
38. Barr CC, Gelender H, Font R. Corneal crystalline deposits associated with dysproteinemia: report of two cases and review of literature. Arch Ophthalmol 1980;98:884–889
39. Eiferman RA, Rodrigues MM. Unusual superficial stromal corneal deposits in benign monoclonal gammopathy. Arch Ophthalmol 1980;98:78–81
40. Miller KH, Green WR, Stark WJ, et al. Immunoprotein deposition in the cornea. Ophthalmology 1980;87:944–950
41. Lewis RA, Falls HF, Troyer DO. Ocular manifestations of hypercupremia associated with multiple myeloma. Arch Ophthalmol 1975;93:1050–1053
42. Smith JW. Ochronosis of the sclera and cornea complicating alkaptonuria: review of the literature and report of four cases. JAMA 1942;120:1282–1288
43. Hatch JL. Hereditary alkaptonuria with ochronosis. Arch Ophthalmol 1959;62: 575–578
44. Garrett EE. Ocular ochronosis with alkaptonuria. Am J Ophthalmol 1963;55: 617–620
45. Rones B. Ochronosis oculi in alkaptonuria. Am J Ophthalmol 1960;49:440–446
46. Wirtschafter JD. The eye in alkaptonuria. Birth Defects 1976;12:279–293
47. Meretoja J. Familial systemic paramyloidosis with lattice dystrophy of the cornea, progressive cranial neuropathy, skin changes and various internal symptoms: a previously unrecognized heritable syndrome. Ann Clin Res 1969;1:314–324
48. Meretoja J. Comparative histopathological and clinical findings in eyes with lattice corneal dystrophy of two types. Ophthalmologica 1972;165:15–37
49. Meretoja J. Genetic aspects of familial amyloidosis with corneal lattice dystrophy and cranial neuropathy. Clin Genet 1973;4:173–185
50. Purcell JJ, Rodrigues MM, Chisti MI, et al. Lattice corneal dystrophy associated with familial systemic amyloidosis (Meretoja's syndrome). Ophthalmology 1983; 90:1512–1517
51. Maury CP, Teppo AM, Karinemi AL, Koeppen AH. Amyloid fibril protein in familial amyloidosis with cranial neuropathy and corneal lattice dystrophy (FAP type IV) is related to transthyretin. Am J Clin Pathol 1988;89:359–364
52. O'Connor GR. Calcific band keratopathy. Trans Am Ophthalmol Soc 1972;70: 58–81
53. Pouliquen Y. Ultrastructure of band keratopathy. Arch Oftalmol (Paris) 1967; 27:149–158
54. Doughman DJ, Olson GA, Nolan S, Hajny RG. Experimental band keratopathy. Arch Ophthalmol 1969;81:264–271
55. Economon JW, Silverstein AM, Zimmerman LE. Band keratopathy in a rabbit colony. Invest Ophthalmol 1963;2:361–368
56. Manschot WA. Ring of Kayser and Fleischer. Ophthalmologica 1956;132:164–166
57. Slovis TL, Dubois RS, Rodgerson DO, Silverman A. The varied manifestations of Wilson's disease. J Pediatr 1971;78:578–584

58. Tso MOM, Fine BS, Thorpe HE. Kayser-Fleischer ring and associated cataract in Wilson's disease. Am J Ophthalmol 1975;79:479–488
59. Scheinberg IH. Wilson's disease. In: Braunwald E et al, eds. Harrison's principles of internal medicine, ed 11. New York: McGraw-Hill, 1987
60. Wiebers DO, Hollenhorst RW, Goldstein NP. The ophthalmological manifestations of Wilson's disease. Mayo Clin Proc 1977;52:409–416
61. Dobyns WB, Goldstein NP, Gordon H. Clinical spectrum of Wilson's disease (hepatolenticular degeneration). Mayo Clin Proc 1979;54:35–42
62. Fleming CR, Dickson ER, Wahner HW, et al. Pigmented rings in non-Wilsonian liver disease. Ann Intern Med 1977;86:285–288
63. Frommer D, Morris J, Sherlock S, et al. Kayser-Fleischer like rings in patients without Wilson's disease. Gastroenterology 1977;72:1331–1335
64. Kaplinsky C, Sternleib I, Javitt N, Rotem Y. Familial cholestatic cirrhosis associated with Kayser-Fleischer rings. Pediatrics 1980;65:782–788
65. Hashimoto A, Maeda Y, Ito H, et al. Corneal chrysiasis: a clinical study in rheumatoid arthritis receiving gold therapy. Arthritis Rheum 1972;15:309–315
66. Kincaid MC, Green WR, Hoover RE, Schenck PH. Ocular chrysiasis. Arch Ophthalmol 1982;100:1791–1794
67. McCormick SA, DiBartolomeo AG, Raju VK, Schwab IR. Ocular chrysiasis. Ophthalmology 1985;92:1432–1435
68. Bron AJ, McLendon BF, Camp AV. Epithelial deposition of gold in the cornea in patients receiving systemic therapy. Am J Ophthalmol 1979;88:354–360
69. Roberts WH, Wolter JR. Ocular chrysiasis. Arch Ophthalmol 1956;56:48–52
70. Rodenhäuser JH, von Behrend T. Type 2 incidence of eye involvement after parenteral gold therapy. Dtsch Med Wochenschr 1969;94:2389–2392
71. Fishman RS, Sunderman RW. Band keratopathy in gout. Arch Ophthalmol 1966;75:367–369
72. Hutchinson J. The relation of certain diseases of the eye to gout. Br Med J 1884;2:995–1000
73. McWilliams JR. Ocular findings in gout. Am J Ophthalmol 1952;35:1778–1783
74. Ferry AP, Safir A, Melikan HE. Ocular abnormalities in patients with gout. Ann Ophthalmol 1985;17:632–635
75. Slansky HH, Kuwabara T. Intranuclear urate crystals in corneal epithelium. Arch Ophthalmol 1968;80:338–344
76. Lüllman H, Lüllmann-Rauch R, Wassermann O. Lipidosis induced by amphophilic cationic drugs. Biochem Pharmacol 1978;27:1103–1108
77. D'Amico DJ, Kenyon KR. Drug-induced lipidoses of the cornea and conjunctiva. Int Ophthalmol 1981;4:67–76
78. François J, Hanssens M, Teuchy H, et al. Ultrastructural findings in macular dystrophy (Groenow type II). Ophthalmic Res 1975;7:80–98
79. Klintworth GK, Smith CF. Abnormalities of proteoglycans and glycoproteins synthesized by corneal organ cultures derived from patients with macular corneal dystrophy. Lab Invest 1983;48:603–612
80. Hassell JR, Newsome DA, Krachmer JH, Rodrigues MM. Macular corneal dystrophy: failure to synthesize a mature keratan sulfate proteoglycan. Proc Natl Acad Sci USA 1980;77:3705–3709
81. Hassell JR, Newsome DA, Nakazawa K, et al. Defective conversion of a glycoprotein precursor to keratan sulfate proteoglycan in macular corneal dystrophy. In: Hawkes S, Wang JL, eds. Extracellular matrix. New York: Academic, 1982
82. Edward DP, Yue BY, Sugar J, et al. Heterogeneity in macular corneal dystrophy. Arch Ophthalmol 1988;106:1579–1583
83. Thonar EJ, Meyer RF, Dennis RF, et al. Absence of normal keratan sulfate in the blood of patients with macular corneal dystrophy. Am J Ophthalmol 1986;102:561–569

84. Melles RB, Schneider JA, Rao NA, Katz B. Spatial and temporal sequence of corneal crystal deposition in nephropathic cystinosis. Am J Ophthalmol 1987; 104:598–604
85. Yamamoto GK, Schulman JD, Schneider JA, Wong VG. Long-term ocular changes in cystinosis: observation in renal transplant recipients. J Pediatr Ophthalmol Strabismus 1979;16:21–25
86. Kaiser-Kupfer MI, Caruso RC, Minkler DS, Gahl WA. Long term ocular manifestations in nephropathic cystinosis. Arch Ophthalmol 1986;104:706–711
87. Katz B, Melles RB, Schneider JA, Rao NA. Corneal thickness in nephropathic cystinosis. Br J Ophthalmol 1989;73:665–668
88. Kaiser-Kupfer MI, Fujikawa L, Kuwabara T, et al. Removal of corneal crystals by topical cysteamine in nephropathic cystinosis. N Engl J Med 1987;316:775–779
89. Kaiser-Kupfer MI, Datiles MB, Gahl WA. Clear graft two years after keratoplasty in nephropathic cystinosis. Am J Ophthalmol 1988;105:318–319
90. Katz B, Melles RB, Schneider JA. Recurrent crystal deposition after keratoplasty in nephropathic cystinosis. Am J Ophthalmol 1987;104:190–191
91. Bienfang DC, Kuwabara T, Pueschel SM. The Richner-Hanhart syndrome: report of a case with associated tyrosinemia. Arch Ophthalmol 1976;94:1133–1137
92. Goldsmith LA, Reed J. Tyrosine-induced eye and skin lesions: a treatable genetic disease. JAMA 1976;236:382–384
93. Colditz PB, Yu JS, Billson FA, et al. Tyrosinaemia II. Med J Aust 1984; 141:244–245
94. Burns RP. Soluble tyrosine aminotransferase deficiency: an unusual cause of corneal ulcers. Am J Ophthalmol 1972;73:400–402
95. Sandberg HO. Bilateral keratopathy in tyrosinosis. Acta Ophthalmol (Copenh) 1975;53:760–764
96. Jaeger W, Gallasch G, Schnyder UW, et al. Herpetiform bilateral epithelial corneal dystrophy caused by tyrosinemia (Richner-Hanhart syndrome). Klin Monatsbl Augenheilkd 1978;173:506–515
97. Charlton KH, Binder PS, Wozniak L, Digby JD. Pseudodendritic keratitis and systemic tyrosinemia. Ophthalmology 1981;88:355–360
98. Gipson IK, Burns RP, Wolfe-Lande JD. Crystals in corneal epithelial lesions of tyrosine-fed rats. Invest Ophthalmol 1975;14:937–942
99. Goldsmith LA, Laberge C. Tyrosinemia and related disorders. In: Scriver CR et al, eds. The metabolic basis of inherited disease, ed 6. New York: McGraw-Hill, 1989
100. Neufeld EF, Muenzer J. The mucopolysaccharidoses. In: Scriver CR et al, eds. The metabolic basis of inherited disease, ed 6. New York: McGraw-Hill, 1989
101. Brown SI, Kuwabara T. Peripheral corneal opacification and skeletal deformities: a newly recognized acid mucopolysaccharidosis simulating rheumatoid arthritis. Arch Ophthalmol 1970;83:667–677
102. Jeanloz RW. The nomenclature of acid mucopolysaccharides. Arthritis Rheum 1960;3:233–237
103. Kenyon KR. Ocular manifestations and pathology of systemic mucopolysaccharidoses. Birth Defects 1976;12:133–153
104. Spranger J. The mucopolysaccharidoses. In: Emery AEH, Rimoin DL, eds. Principles and practice of medical genetics. New York: Churchill Livingstone, 1983:1339
105. Van Hoof F, Hers HG. The abnormalities of lysosomal enzymes in mucopolysaccharidoses. Eur J Biochem 1968;7:34–44
106. Nolan CM, Sly CS. I-cell disease and pseudo-Hurler polydystrophy: disorders of lysosomal enzyme phosphorylation and localization. In Scriver CR et al, eds. The metabolic basis of inherited disease, ed 6. New York: McGraw-Hill, 1989
107. Luchsinger U, Bühler EM, Méhes K, Hirt HR. I-cell disease. N Engl J Med 1970;282:1374–1375

108. Lightbody J, Wiesmann U, Hadorn B, Herschkowitz N. I-cell disease: multiple lysosomal-enzyme defect. Lancet 1971;1:451
109. Borit A, Sugarman GI, Spencer WH. Ocular involvement in I-cell disease (mucolipidosis II) light and electron-microscopic findings. Albrecht von Graefes Arch Klin Exp Ophthalmol 1976;198:25–32
110. Libert J, Van Hoof F, Farriaux JP, Toussaint D. Ocular findings in I-cell disease (mucolipidosis type II). Am J Ophthalmol 1977;83:617–628
111. Kelly TE, Thomas GH, Taylor HA, et al. Mucolipidosis III (pseudo-Hurler polydystrophy): clinical and laboratory studies in a series of 12 patients. Johns Hopkins Med J 1975;137:156–175
112. Traboulsi EI, Maumenee IH. Ophthalmic findings in mucolipidosis III (pseudo-Hurler polydystrophy). Am J Ophthalmol 1986;102:592–597
113. Kenyon KR, Sensenbrenner JA. Mucolipidosis II (I-cell disease): ultrastructural observations of conjunctiva and sclera. Invest Ophthalmol 1971;10:555–567
114. Quigley HA, Goldberg MF. Conjunctival ultrastructure in mucolipidosis 3 (pseudo-Hurler polydystrophy). Invest Ophthalmol 1971;10:568–580
115. Hashimoto K, Lieberman P, Lamkin N. Angiokeratoma corporis diffusum (Fabry's disease). Arch Dermatol 1976;112:1416–1423
116. Karr WJ Jr. Fabry's disease (angiokeratoma corporis diffusum universale). Am J Med 1959;7:829–835
117. Grace EV. Diffuse angiokeratosis (Fabry's disease). Am J Ophthalmol 1966;62: 139–145
118. Sher NA, Letson RD, Desnick RJ. The ocular manifestations in Fabry's disease. Arch Ophthalmol 1979;97:671–676
119. Spaeth GL, Frost P. Fabry's disease: its ocular manifestations. Arch Ophthalmol 1965;74:760–769
120. Franceschetti AT. Fabry's disease: ocular manifestations. Birth Defects 1976; 12:195–208
121. Weingeist TA, Blodi FC. Fabry's disease: ocular findings in a female carrier. A light and electron microscopic study. Arch Ophthalmol 1971;85:169–176
122. Font RL, Fine BS. Ocular pathology in Fabry's disease. Am J Ophthalmol 1973; 73:419–430
123. François J, Hanssens M, Teuchy H. Corneal ultrastructural changes in Fabry's disease. Ophthalmologica 1978;176:313–330
124. Frost P, Tamala Y, Spaeth GL. Fabry's disease—glycolipid lipidosis: histochemical and electron microscopic studies of two cases. Am J Med 1966;40:618–627
125. Riegel EM, Pokorny KS, Friedman AH, et al. Ocular pathology of Fabry's disease in a hemizygous male following renal transplantation. Surv Ophthalmol 1982; 26:247–252
126. Mosher HW, Prensky AL, Wolfe JG, Rosman NP. Farber's lipogranulomatosis. Report of a case and demonstration of an excess of free ceramide and ganglioside. Am J Med 1969;47:869–890
127. Ozaki H, Mizutani M, Hayashi H, et al. Farber's disease (disseminated lipogranulomatosis): the first case reported in Japan. Acta Med Okayama 1978;32:69–79
128. Zetterstrom R. Disseminated lipogranulomatosis (Farber's disease). Acta Paediatr Scand 1958;47:501–508
129. Zarbin MA, Green WR, Moser HW, Morton SJ. Farber's disease. Light and electron microscopic study of the eye. Arch Ophthalmol 1985;103:73–80
130. Goldberg MF, Cotlier E, Fichenscher LG, et al. Macular cherry-red spot, corneal clouding, and beta-galactosidase deficiency: clinical, biochemical, and electron microscopic study of a new autosomal recessive storage disease. Arch Intern Med 1971;128:387–398
131. Libert J, Van Hoof F, Tonduer M. Fucosidosis: ultrastructural study of conjunctiva and skin and enzyme analysis of tears. Invest Ophthalmol 1976;15:626–639

132. Hoshino M, O'Brien TP, McDonnell JM, et al. Fucosidosis: ultrastructural study of the eye in an adult. Graefes Arch Clin Exp Ophthalmol 1989;227:162–171
133. Cibis GW, Harris DJ, Chapman AL, Tripathi RC. Mucolipidosis I. Arch Ophthalmol 1983;101:933–939
134. Emery JM, Greene WR, Wyllie RG, et al. Gm_1-gangliosidosis: ocular and pathological manifestations. Arch Ophthalmol 1971;85:177–187
135. Arbisser AI, Murphree AL, Garcia CA, Howell RR. Ocular findings in mannosidosis. Am J Ophthalmol 1976;82:465–471
136. Borrone C, Gatti R, Trias X, et al. Fucosidosis: clinical, biochemical, immunologic, and genetic studies in two new cases. J Pediatr 1974;84:727–730
137. Snyder RO, Carlow TJ, Ledman J, Wenger DA. Ocular findings in fucosidosis. Birth Defects 1976;12:241–251

Systemic Associations of Scleritis

Kim N. Hakin, F.R.C.S., F.C.Ophth.
Peter G. Watson, F.R.C.S., F.C.Ophth.

Scleral inflammation from whatever cause is associated with readily detectable changes in the visible coats of the episclera and conjunctiva. These changes may be localized to the sclera or may be part of a generalized systemic vasculitis, often as a late manifestation of some connective tissue disease. The clinical manifestations of an immunological assault on blood vessels depends on many factors, including the nature of immune response to the initial insult, the nature and severity of the resulting inflammation, and the genetic makeup of the patient. This means that inflammation of the sclera can occur in what, at first sight, appears to be a bewildering number of disorders. Sometimes it is clear why the sclera has become involved—for example, following trauma or with chronic infection in patients with immunologically induced disorders—but at other times, there are no obvious precipitating factors. However, there are distinct clinical patterns of disease that will help to distinguish those who have localized disease that will not damage the eye from those who have severe disease that will undoubtedly harm the eye unless treated effectively and early in the course of the condition. There are also distinguishing features within the severe disorders that will help to differentiate the underlying systemic conditions, of importance when deciding a specific therapy. These all depend on very careful clinical observation of the sclera, cornea, and visible vascular networks [1].

Clinical Manifestations and Pathological Changes Found in Scleral Disease

Episcleritis

Typically occurring in young women, episcleritis is a common, benign, recurrent inflammation of the episclera, the loose connective tissue layer overlying the sclera, including Tenon's capsule. It presents as a watery, uncomfortable, red eye; the absence of severe pain and scleral swelling and the maintenance of the normal radial vascular configuration usually distinguishes the

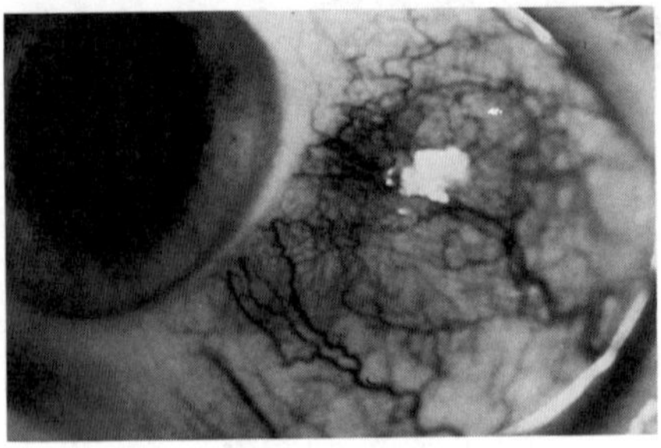

Figure 1 *Nodular episcleritis. The superficial nodule involves the episcleral tissue only and will respond to local steroid therapy.*

condition from scleritis, although in some cases this may be difficult. In simple episcleritis, there is diffuse edema in the region of vascular congestion, usually in the interpalpebral region. In nodular episcleritis, in which one or more nodules form, the disease tends to run a protracted course. When examining the patient, it is important to ensure that the underlying sclera has retained its normal contours as the more severe nodular scleritis may require more aggressive therapy and may even develop rapidly into a necrotizing scleritis (Figs 1, 2). Episcleritis is usually self-limiting, requiring no treatment, although a short course of topical steroids will hasten resolution. There is no regular association with any systemic disorder, although gout was detected in 7% of patients in one series [2].

Scleritis

Scleritis is a more serious disorder than episcleritis. It presents with deep, severe, periorbital pain radiating to the temple and jaw, typically waking the patient at night. Approximately 50% of patients have an underlying systemic disorder. Because of the peculiarities in the distribution of the vascular supply to the anterior segment of the eye, which leaves segments poorly perfused or with oscillations of arterial blood, scleritis is more common anterior to the equator [3, 4]. However, it does occur posteriorly, causing considerable diagnostic difficulty.

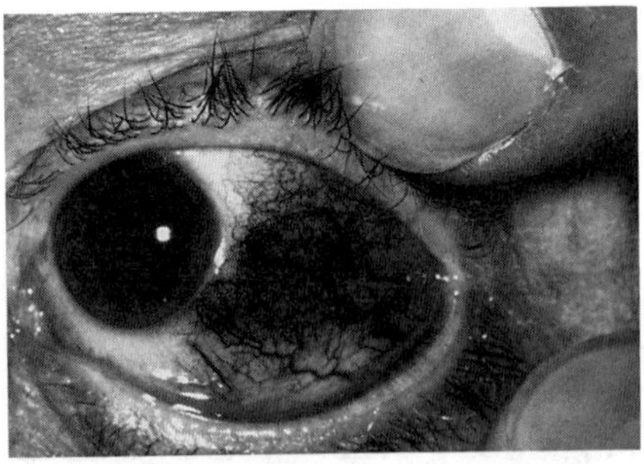

Figure 2 *Intense localized redness in nodular scleritis in a patient with relapsing polychondritis. The deep vessels are displaced over the nodule (see Fig 1). This requires systemic therapy.*

Anterior Scleritis Anterior scleritis is classified as diffuse, nodular, and necrotizing, with or without inflammation [5]. Diffuse anterior scleritis is the most benign form. One-fourth of patients have some systemic connective tissue disorder, usually rheumatoid arthritis. There is an intense violaceous vascular congestion, which may involve a small area or the whole of the anterior segment. Slit-lamp examination reveals swelling and injection of the sclera, with an overlying episcleritis, and a disturbance of the normal radial pattern of the superficial episcleral vessels, with closure of capillaries and replacement by vascular loops derived from the capillary network, together with new, abnormal vascular channels that appear both to feed and drain the affected area. After the acute episode has resolved, the new vasculature persists. The sclera may appear to be translucent, taking on a gray-blue discoloration, which is not due to scleral loss or thinning but to rearrangement of the collagen fibers within the sclera (Fig 3).

Discrete scleral nodules are present in nodular scleritis. They are deep red due to intense vascular congestion, are immobile and exquisitely tender, and are quite separate from the overlying edematous episclera (see Fig 2). Multiple nodules may be confluent or, occasionally, discrete. If the center of a nodule becomes avascular, necrosis usually ensues. Uveitis and glaucoma are rare in scleritis. If they occur, it may be assumed that the trabecular tissue or ciliary body is affected by the granulomatous process.

Necrotizing scleritis is an uncommon form of scleritis but is potentially sight-threatening. It can occur with or without accompanying inflammation. When associated with systemic disease, it is always associated with systemic vasculitis, which is life-threatening. Necrotizing scleritis with inflammation typically occurs in people between the ages of 30 and 60 and is bilateral in more than half the cases. Most patients will not have had any previous scleral inflammation. It usually presents with intense pain and discomfort, which may appear to be out of proportion to the clinical signs. Careful examination of the vascular pattern will reveal areas of poor or absent perfusion and may also show yellow-white avascular areas of episcleral, and sometimes conjunctival, tissue overlying an area of scleral edema. There is intense inflammation at the edges of the lesion which, if untreated, tends to progress circumferentially, leaving behind white or translucent, avascular, thinned areas of sclera (Fig 4). Progression does not usually extend to behind the equator. Severe intraocular complications are almost inevitable once the cornea has been encircled by scle-

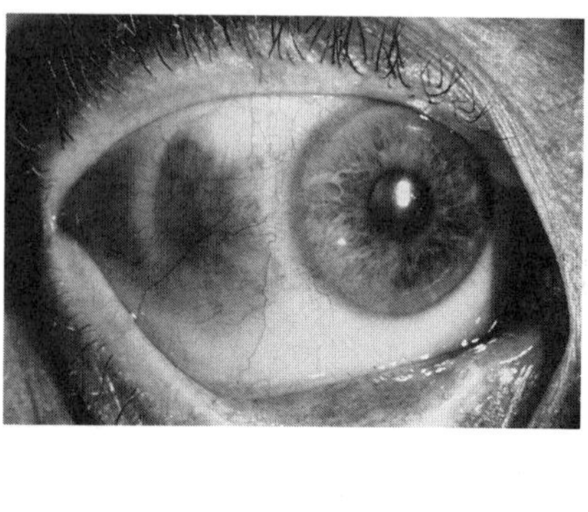

Figure 3 *Translucent sclera that ensued after treatment of scleritis in a patient with relapsing polychondritis. The scleritis in this condition is very resistant to treatment. Patient required "pulsed" steroid therapy and prolonged systemic steroids and cyclosporine to control the condition.*

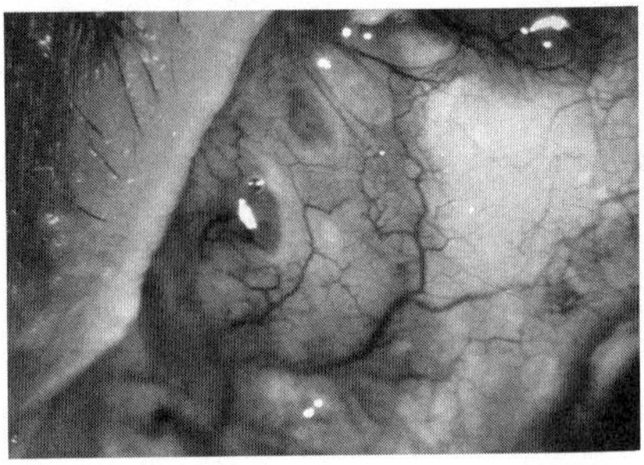

Figure 4 *Necrotizing scleritis with inflammation in a 58-year-old man with rheumatoid arthritis of acute onset 3 years previously. Patient also had vasculitic lesions on the hands and elbows. The eye was very painful, and both the cornea and sclera are affected by the vasculitic process, which has led to obliteration of the capillary nets of the episclera and limbus.*

ritis. The disease may follow an insidious course, progressing slowly over several months or very acutely over several days, in which case the disease is often bilateral and associated with an exacerbation of a systemic vasculitis. Scleral necrosis may result in the exposure of large areas of choroid or ciliary muscle, which is covered by only a thin layer of conjunctiva. Even if the intraocular pressure is raised, perforation is unusual in the absence of trauma.

Necrotizing scleritis without inflammation (scleromalacia perforans) usually occurs in elderly women, is generally bilateral, and is nearly always associated with long-standing rheumatoid disease. It produces a painless insidious necrosis of the sclera and, thus, patients are usually asymptomatic. Areas of sclera and episclera become thinned and avascular, without any surrounding inflammation, and may become sequestered from surrounding normal tissue (Fig 5). Despite large areas of exposed uveal tissue, staphylomas do not occur, although such eyes are very vulnerable to mild trauma. If perforation does occur and the sclera is not repaired, then phthisis bulbi results.

Posterior Scleritis Posterior scleritis is an inflammation of the sclera behind the equator, which may or may not be associated with anterior scleritis. It is far more common than previously recognized. Although it typically presents with pain, visual loss, and proptosis with limited range of ocular movement, the mode of presentation can be very variable, so that the diagnosis may be frequently missed or delayed [6, 7]. As a result of the swollen sclera and episclera, a wide variety of fundal signs may be seen: disc swelling, exudative

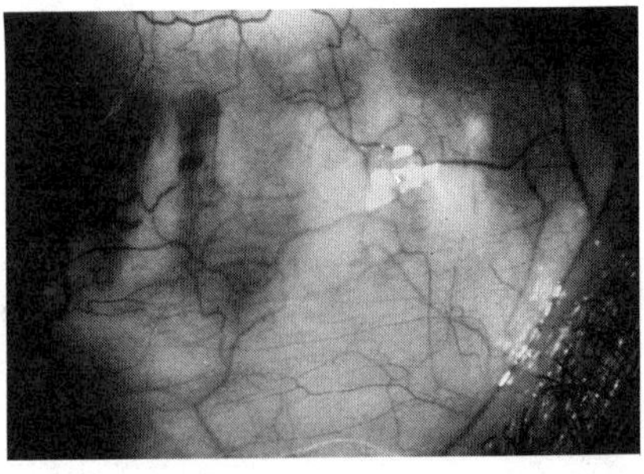

Figure 5 *Necrotizing scleritis without inflammation* (scleromalacia perforans, *a term that should be reserved for patients with this condition). This 62-year-old woman had crippling rheumatoid arthritis for 20 years. She noticed, by chance, that the eye was changing color, though there was no pain or inflammation. This lesion is due to infarction of the arterial supply of the anterior segment and, if it is not accompanied by an inflammatory response, does not need to be treated.*

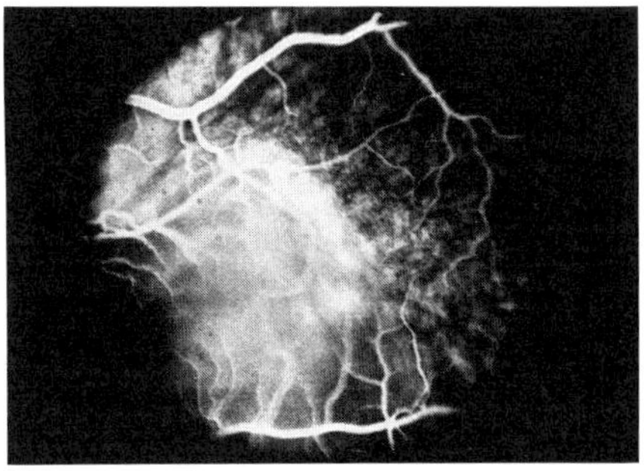

Figure 6 *Posterior scleritis. This diagnosis is often missed because of the multiple presenting features. It is not always painful. Patient is a 26-year-old woman who presented with deteriorating vision and discomfort but no severe pain. She was found to have choroidal folds, focal leaking points from the choroid, and mild disc edema. B-scan ultrasonography revealed a thickened posterior sclera that rapidly resolved with systemic treatment with nonsteroidal antiinflammatory agents. In this case, no systemic disorder was detected.*

retinal detachment (which may be mistaken for a choroidal melanoma), macular edema, choroidal detachment, choroidal folds, and pigment epithelial detachments (Fig 6). Glaucoma can occur, either due to angle closure or as a result of inflammation affecting the trabecular meshwork. There is an associated systemic disorder in more than 50% of cases. B-scan ultrasonography, which demonstrates thickening of the posterior coats of the eye, is the most effective tool for diagnosing this condition.

Clinical and Histological Findings Anterior segment fluorescein angiography (ASFA) is useful for demonstrating the vascular changes that occur in scleritis and for differentiating those patients who may have vascular closure and therefore require intensive therapy [8]. In episcleritis, there is greatly increased vascular flow but the vascular pattern remains unchanged and, after resolution of the acute episode, there are no signs to suggest any previous inflammation. While in some eyes with anterior diffuse or nodular scleritis, the fluorescein vascular pattern may be similar to that seen in episcleritis, in others there are marked changes in the angiographic appearance. Despite being clinically congested, little or no blood is being carried in the vessels; the filling pattern of the vessels is distorted, with the opening of abnormal anastomoses, giving rise to shunt or bypass vessels. If the capillaries and small arterioles fill at all, they fill slowly, and the transit time is greatly reduced (Fig 7). The vascular anomalies persist after the inflammation has subsided, and the patent vessels remain permeable for a long period after resolution of the

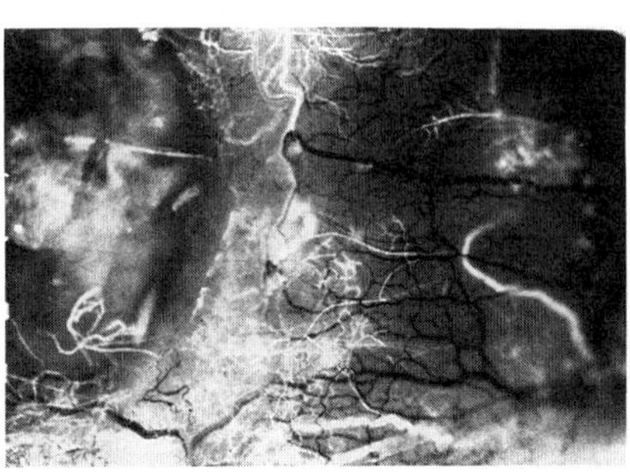

Figure 7 *Anterior segment fluorescein angiography in a 60-year-old man with severe systemic vasculitis. There was a peripheral corneal gutter but no scleral inflammation. The capillary network is unperfused and remained so throughout the sequence. Anterior segment angiography is of value in patients who might be developing necrotizing scleritis and for assessing the response to treatment in patients with limbal leakage, as in Wegener's granulomatosis.*

acute attack. Necrosis occurs as a result of the intense inflammatory reaction, which is often found in an area of poor vascular perfusion. Scleritis with inflammation usually involves the venules but, in scleromalacia perforans, the arterioles become occluded, resulting in infarction and sequestration of scleral tissue that is gradually removed. The subsequent replacement by fibrous tissue is sparse but sufficient to keep the globe intact.

The main histological finding in scleritis is a chronic granuloma [9]. In necrotizing scleritis, there is central necrosis and a surrounding cellular infiltrate of plasma cells, lymphocytes (predominantly T cells), and macrophages that may aggregate into giant cells. The appearance of neutrophils is a late feature of disease and is found only in areas of necrotic sclera. The granuloma is surrounded by old and new vessels, many of which are thrombosed and cuffed, characteristic of a vasculitis.

It must be appreciated that inflammatory changes are progressing in tissues distant from the manifest granuloma, even in those areas that appear normal by light microscopy [10]. Electron microscopy reveals active changes within the scleral stromal fibrocytes, together with changes in the proteoglycan surrounding the collagen fibrils of the sclera, which are unraveled and eventually resorbed. As the clinically abnormal tissue is approached, a cellular infiltrate, chiefly of plasma cells and lymphocytes, can be observed. ASFA may demonstrate vascular closure in these clinically normal areas of sclera.

The presence of a vasculitis suggests an underlying immune complex (type III) reaction, in which the vascular response is the result of conjugation of antigen-antibody within and outside the vessel wall, with subsequent activation of complement. A recent study of the distribution of complement within the sclera found that, with the exception of C1, complement levels were higher in posterior sclera than anterior sclera, together with higher levels of albumin and immunoglobulin, indicating that posterior sclera, by virtue of its underlying choroid, has a greater and more evenly distributed vascular supply [11]. C1 is the recognition unit of the classical complement pathway, and it may be that in scleritis caused by immune complex deposition, the raised levels may allow easier initiation of the complement cascade at areas of reduced vascular flow. In the anterior sclera, these occur at the watershed zones between the supplies of the anterior ciliary arteries, at the 10 and 2 o'clock positions above and 4 and 8 o'clock positions below, and at the posterior ciliary arteries via perforating vessels [3].

Scleral inflammation probably starts as a result of a local insult, such as mild infection or trauma, which damages the vessels and induces an immune response that persists. This develops into an autoimmune process with a local vasculitis, tissue hypoxia, and activation of complement. In certain systemic vasculitic disorders, circulating immune complexes probably affect the scleral vessels directly, setting up a local inflammatory response, particularly if these vessels have been altered through a previous minor insult.

Pathological evidence of immune complexes has been demonstrated in some cases, chiefly in those with an associated systemic vasculitis, but it is not a universal finding [12]. Also, complement activation should result in the accumulation of neutrophils; the absence of these cells in early disease does not support the idea of immune complex perpetuation of the disease. The presence of granuloma formation suggests an underlying delayed hypersensitivity (type IV) reaction, the result of cellular immunity, chiefly involving T lymphocytes. T cells have indeed been demonstrated to be present in large numbers; macrophages may be dealing with local antigens and presenting them to the T cells, which are then activated locally.

■ Systemic Associations

The pathological changes found in scleral disease are the same as, or very similar to, those found in a large number of connective tissue disorders, which in part of their clinical course present with a vasculitis. Although scleritis is a relatively rare extraarticular manifestation of these disorders, representing between 6 and 11% of those affected, it may be the presenting feature. The most common connective tissue disorder associated with scleritis is rheumatoid arthritis. Some of the ocular conditions are to be found only in association with a particular connective tissue disease, but it is important to recognize that many of the others are common to any of the other vasculitides.

Rheumatoid Arthritis

The incidence of scleritis in patients with rheumatoid arthritis varies from 0.15 to 6.3%; the largest series of 4,210 patients gave an incidence of 0.67% [13]. Conversely, the incidence of rheumatoid arthritis in patients presenting with scleritis is 30%.

It is a chronic, multisystem, inflammatory disorder that predominantly affects the musculoskeletal system, characteristically presenting with an insidious, symmetrical polyarthritis. This may be accompanied by constitutional symptoms such as fever, malaise, and loss of appetite. Occasionally, the disease may have an acute onset. The small joints of the hand and wrist (with the exception of the distal interphalangeal joints) are usually involved initially, with more proximal joints affected as the disease progresses. Progressive joint destruction leads to limitation of movement and, in certain cases, subluxation as a result of stretching of the joint capsule and laxity of the ligaments.

Subcutaneous rheumatoid nodules occur in one-third of patients and are found at pressure points, typically on the extensor surface of the forearm. A vasculitis may occur in rheumatoid arthritis, often at the stage where the articular manifestations are inactive. The vasculitis affects all sizes of vessels, ranging from the large arterial trunks to small arteries in nailfolds and the arterioles of the sclera. It may result in a pleurisy, pericarditis, or myocarditis, although these are sometimes asymptomatic, only to be found incidentally on radiography or at postmortem. A central or peripheral neuropathy can occur, either as a result of a vasculitis or secondary to physical compression caused by the joint deformities.

It is clear from what has already been discussed that there will be little or nothing to distinguish the scleritis seen in rheumatoid arthritis from any other disease, except that necrotizing scleritis without surrounding inflammation (scleromalacia perforans), in which there is infarction of scleral tissue, rarely occurs in any condition other than rheumatoid arthritis. There are, however, corneal changes, the appearance of which (with or without accompanying scle-

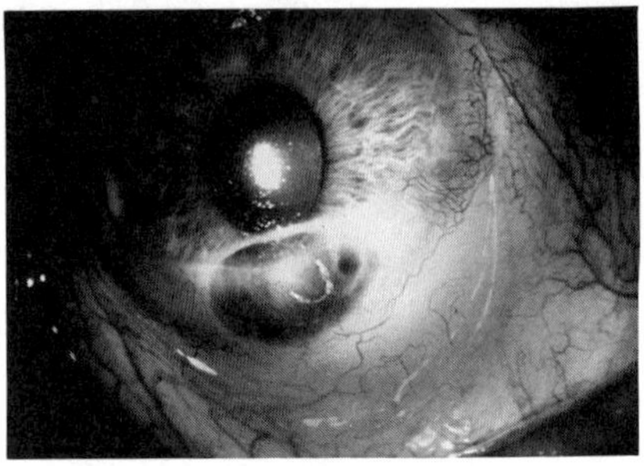

Figure 8 *Peripheral corneal thinning in a patient with long-standing rheumatoid arthritis. This corneal change appears without pain or inflammation and was associated with total vascular obliteration in the region of the thinning.*

ritis) is much more common in rheumatoid arthritis than in any other condition. In long-standing rheumatoid arthritis, there is a progressive attenuation of the limbal vascular supply and a consequent reduction in peripheral corneal nutrition. This leads to a change that, because of its appearance, is best described as a *contact lens* cornea, in which the center of the cornea remains of normal thickness but there is marked thinning of the peripheral cornea without a change in transparency [14]. These corneas, which never cause problems, have to be distinguished from the corneal guttering or melting that accompanies an immunologically induced scleritis or limbitis (Fig 8). This type of melting occurs as a result of limbal vasculitis and so can be seen in other connective tissue disorders. Central corneal necrosis can occur but only when there is severe destructive change involving the whole anterior segment of the eye.

Other than scleritis, the major ocular manifestation of rheumatoid arthritis is keratoconjunctivitis sicca (KCS), in which there is reduced quantity and quality of lacrimal secretion. When this is associated with similar changes in the salivary glands and mucosal glands of the upper respiratory tract and genital tract, it is Sjögren's syndrome.

Rheumatoid arthritis is characterized by the presence of rheumatoid factors. These are autoantibodies directed against antigenic sites in the F_c portion of the heavy chain of immunoglobulin (Ig) molecules. They may be IgG, IgM, IgA, or IgE, but laboratory tests generally detect only the IgM factor. Positive serological studies are present in 80% of patients with rheumatoid arthritis and confirm the diagnosis, especially if in a titer of more than 1:80.

The etiology and role of rheumatoid factors are not known, but it is believed that they are involved in the formation of immune complexes. They are not specific to rheumatoid arthritis (they may be found in other conditions such as systemic lupus erythematosus) and, although they do not parallel disease activity, they do correlate with extraarticular manifestations. IgE-containing immune complexes have recently been identified, and these appear to correlate with disease activity.

The vasculitis of rheumatoid arthritis, as with scleritis, is believed to be the result of immune complex deposition in, or just outside, vessel walls, activating complement; raised levels of circulating immune complexes tend to be associated with low levels of complement. A common role for immune complexes is supported by the fact that a systemic vasculitis, or other extraarticular manifestation of rheumatoid arthritis, is nearly always found in rheumatoid patients with scleritis. Rao and colleagues [12], in a histopathological study of 41 cases of scleritis, describe in those cases associated with systemic autoimmune disorders areas of zonal scleral inflammation originating from adjacent episcleral and uveal tissue, in a pattern that they believed was compatible with an immune complex–mediated vasculitis.

Immune complex reactions, however, clearly are not the only pathological process involved in rheumatoid arthritis. Early pathological changes in the joints are of an acute synovitis with an intense lymphocytic and plasma cell infiltrate. Most of the lymphocytes are T cells of the CD4+/helper phenotype [15, 16]. An increase in the CD4:CD8 ratio in peripheral blood and bone marrow, and in the percentage of T cells expressing major histocompatibility complex (MHC) class II antigens (encoded by HLA-D antigens) has been reported [17, 18]. There is an association of rheumatoid arthritis with HLA-DR4 and -Dw4, supporting the idea that cellular immunity also plays a role in the development of rheumatoid arthritis [19, 20].

Juvenile Polyarthritis

Juvenile chronic arthritis is diagnosed on the presence of an arthritis of more than 3 months' duration, commencing before the sixteenth birthday. It does not include the arthritides associated with collagen disorders, trauma, neoplasia, or infection, or the HLA-B27-related arthropathies such as ankylosing spondylitis or Reiter's syndrome. Three subgroups of juvenile chronic arthritis are generally recognized: systemic onset, polyarticular onset, and pauciarticular onset [21]. Approximately 25% of the polyarticular-onset group are seropositive for IgM rheumatoid factor and follow a clinical path similar to that of adults with rheumatoid arthritis. The predominant ocular manifestation of juvenile arthritis is a chronic anterior uveitis, which is accompanied by minimal inflammation and which occurs in association with pauciarticular arthritis, usually in girls who are seropositive for antinuclear factor [22]. Should a child with arthritis develop scleritis or episcleritis, however, he or she is almost always from the polyarticular group and is usually seropositive for rheumatoid factor. The scleritis is usually of the diffuse or, occasionally, the nodular variety. It is clinically indistinguishable from a scleritis due to any other cause except that it may be more difficult to see the scleral swelling because of the thick episclera. Children with the systemic form of the disease (Still's disease) do not develop eye problems; those with pauciarticular arthritis do not develop scleritis. The limbal tissue does, however, swell in some with active uveitis.

Systemic Lupus Erythematosus

Systemic lupus erythematosus (SLE) is an uncommon disease, predominantly affecting women (90% of cases). The prevalence varies with different populations, blacks being more frequently affected than whites. There is an association with HLA-B8 in whites and HLA-A1 in blacks. The basic pathological process is a vasculitis; hence the widespread organ involvement.

SLE usually presents with nonspecific symptoms such as fever, weight loss, fatigue, and an arthromyalgia, although a destructive arthritis is rare. Skin disease occurs in 80% of patients, the classical butterfly rash extending across the bridge of the nose to the malar areas being present in approximately half the patients at diagnosis. A cutaneous vasculitis, usually in the forearms and fingers, and alopecia of all the body hair, may occur. Discoid lupus refers to the raised, erythematous, well-demarcated lesions usually found on the face, and less commonly on the trunk and arms, and may occur in isolation. Vasculitis commonly results in glomerulonephritis, which is particularly serious if of the proliferative form, and can also affect the heart, lung, and central nervous system. Although almost every ocular structure may be affected, the most common manifestation is of a retinal vascular disease (chiefly affecting the arterioles), which is usually associated with active cerebral lupus. Conjunctivitis, KCS, and epithelial keratitis also occur.

Scleritis is not uncommon and is almost always of the diffuse or nodular variety. It is resistant to treatment until the systemic disease is brought under control with systemic steroids or immunosuppressive agents. Surprisingly, even though ASFA shows a limbal vasculitis, in these patients the changes are not destructive but are characterized by lipid deposition in the cornea resulting from leaking limbal capillaries.

SLE is characterized by a variety of immunological features exhibited in the peripheral blood. Detection of the presence of antinuclear antibody factor (ANA) is a sensitive but not very specific test for SLE. However, ANA is present in 95% of cases and so provides a useful screening test.

Lupus cells are present in approximately 80% of lupus patients (and occasionally in patients with other connective tissue diseases, rheumatoid arthritis, and chronic liver disease). The lupus (LE) cell is a polymorphonuclear leukocyte that has engulfed nuclear material, itself extruded from a leukocyte that has been destroyed by the penetration of antinuclear antibody [23].

The presence of antibodies to double-stranded DNA is a more specific test for SLE, the levels generally reflecting disease activity. A wide range of autoantibodies is, in fact, detectable in lupus patients, including those to single-stranded DNA, cardiolipin, histones, ribonucleoprotein, and adenosine diphosphate–ribose [24]. The presence of antibodies to phospholipid appears to be a risk factor for the development of occlusive vascular disease in SLE [25].

The principal pathological finding in SLE is a vasculitis of small arteries with fibrinoid necrosis of the vessel walls. High levels of circulating and tissue immune complexes are commonly found. Immunopathological studies on eyes from patients with SLE, obtained at autopsy, have demonstrated by direct fluorescence a pattern suggestive of immune complex deposits in the walls of blood vessels of the conjunctiva, ciliary body, retina, choroid, and sclera [26, 27]. Although it would seem likely that these immune complexes are the result of the autoantibodies combining with antigen, this has been difficult to prove.

Sunlight, infection, and a number of drugs including hydralazine, procainamide, isoniazid, sulfonamides, and oral contraceptives, are known to trigger the disease. Activity may increase in pregnancy. Examination of the amino acid sequences in the hypervariable segments (idiotypes) of the anti-DNA antibodies has revealed a constant idiotype, named *16/6,* which is present in the serum and kidney biopsies of many patients with SLE [28]. It is believed that this may be pathogenic, as procainamide has been shown to induce increased production of this idiotype and immunization of previously healthy mice with an antibody with this idiotype leads to a lupus type disorder [29].

The cellular immune system also plays a role: Decreased levels of interleukin-2 and reduced cytotoxic and natural killer cell activity are known to occur [30, 31].

Wegener's Granulomatosis

Wegener's granulomatosis (WG) is a multisystem disease initially regarded as a variant of polyarteritis nodosa but then classified separately because of its distinct clinical pattern. It is diagnosed on the basis of three pathological criteria: necrotizing granulomas of the respiratory tract, a generalized necrotizing vasculitis, and necrotizing glomerulonephritis [32]. It is most common in the fourth and fifth decade and, until the introduction of systemic immunosuppressive therapy (corticosteroids and cyclophosphamide), was nearly always fatal, usually due to renal involvement, with a rapidly progressive course over several months. The association with HLA antigens B8 and DR2 and the reported incidence in several members of one family indicates a genetic predisposition.

The nasal passages and upper respiratory tract are virtually always involved, producing facial and sinus pain and nasal discharge, and may progress to nasal septal ulceration and perforation. There are usually associated systemic symptoms such as night sweats, weakness, weight loss, and arthralgia. Serous otitis media with eustachian tube blockage is a common otological manifestation. Pulmonary disease causing cough, hemoptysis, and dyspnea frequently occurs.

Glomerulonephritis is said to occur in approximately 80% of patients and, once started, signals the onset of progressive disease. Unlike polyarteritis, hypertension-associated renal disease is uncommon, but the cutaneous vasculitis, represented by purpura, ulceration, vesicles, or nodules, is common.

Ocular manifestations, which may be the first sign of WG, are present in up to 50% of cases. Extraocular disease, such as nasolacrimal duct obstruction, proptosis, or extraocular muscle involvement, generally occurs secondary to contiguous granulomatous sinus disease. The most common ocular complication is proptosis due to retrobulbar granulomatous infiltration, which is often bilateral and can present acutely [33, 34]. The changes seen in the anterior segment of the globe, which are the result of the fulminating vasculitis, are so typical as to be diagnostic of WG. As they can occur in isolation at a very early stage in this systemic disease, it is very important to recognize them so that appropriate management can be given to the patient to prevent progression of the disease. The granulomatous changes involve conjunctiva, episclera, and sclera (Fig 9), but rarely cause a uveitis unless the ciliary body becomes directly involved. Characteristically, the patient presents with the symptoms of a scleritis—severe pain in the eye and head, watering of the eye, and localized redness of the globe. On examination, the inflammatory changes can be seen to involve all layers of the coats of the eye, together with a raised granulomatous mass which, in the earliest stages, is best observed with the red-free light on the slit lamp. This method of examination shows the extent of infiltration under and through the conjunctiva and episclera. If the lesion is adjacent to

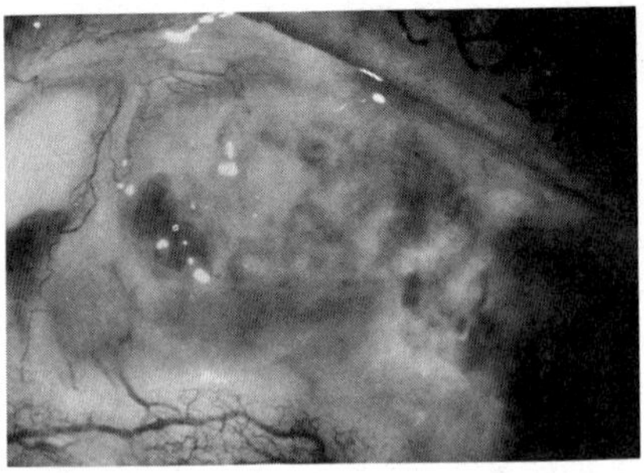

Figure 9 *Wegener's granulomatosis, in which all the layers of the coats of the eye become involved in the destructive granuloma. This lesion healed completely following treatment with systemic steroid and cyclophosphamide.*

the limbus, careful observation of the limbal arcade of vessels will show that the arcade is broken and that the vessels leak profusely. Adjacent to this leakage, the tissue of both cornea and sclera is being destroyed (Fig 10). These small areas become confluent, and a gutter appears that involves limbal tissue. This transgression of the limbus by a destructive change is seen only in WG and polyarteritis nodosa. Disease control with steroids and cyclophosphamide, or occasionally with plasma exchange, can be monitored very closely by observation of the limbal vessels, which cease to leak once treatment is adequate.

Vasculitis and granulomatous inflammation with extensive necrosis are the characteristic pathological findings of WG [35]. Biopsy of granulomatous tissue in the nose and sinuses is often helpful [36]. The necrosis typically is basophilic with serpiginous borders and is surrounded by granulomatous inflammation. Multinucleate giant cells and microabscesses consisting of neutrophils, lymphocytes, and plasma cells may be found. Renal biopsy commonly demonstrates a proliferative focal glomerulonephritis with necrosis and thrombosis of individual loops; sometimes all the glomeruli are destroyed.

The cause of WG is not known, although bacterial and viral infections can induce relapses [37]. The diagnosis of WG has previously been based on clinical and histopathological findings. An autoimmune process has long been suspected on the basis of response to cyclophosphamide and plasma exchange and the presence of circulating immune complexes, rheumatoid factor, and antinuclear antibodies. The discovery, by indirect immunofluorescence, in serum of patients with WG, microscopic polyarteritis nodosa, and segmental necrotizing glomerulonephritis, of a circulating IgG autoantibody against in-

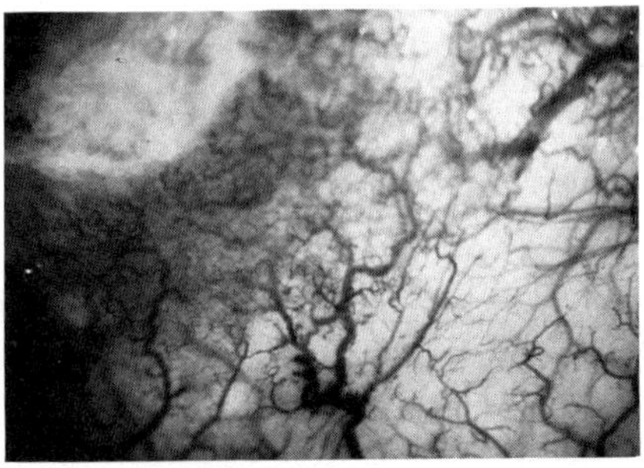

Figure 10 *Wegener's granulomatosis. The granulomatous process has involved both the cornea and sclera, a condition that occurs only in polyarteritis nodosa and Wegener's granulomatosis.*

tracytoplasmic extranuclear components of neutrophils—the antineutrophil cytoplasmic antibody (ANCA; synonym, *anticytoplasmic antibody* [ACPA])—has supported the autoimmune pathogenesis and provided a specific immunological marker for a systemic vasculitis. ANCAs are nearly always present in this condition [38]. The antibody levels correlate with disease activity, but it is not clear whether they are a cause or an effect of the disease. Two types of ANCA can be demonstrated, according to the pattern of immunofluorescence produced. C-ANCAs display uniform fine granular staining of the cytoplasm; the antigen is believed usually to be a proteinase. P-ANCAs display perinuclear staining and appear usually to be directed against myeloperoxidase or elastase [39–41]. It has been suggested that P-ANCA is associated with renal disease and C-ANCA with lung and sinus disease [42].

Antiendothelial cell antibodies (AECA) have been detected more recently in systemic vasculitides and appear to be markers in a similar manner to ANCA [43].

Polyarteritis Nodosa

Polyarteritis nodosa (PAN) is an uncommon disorder that is characterized by a necrotizing vasculitis of medium-sized and small arteries and may affect virtually any organ in the body. It occurs more commonly in men, usually in the fifth and sixth decade of life. It may present with constitutional symptoms such as malaise, fever, and weight loss, or symptoms arising from specific organ involvement, such as the nephrotic syndrome or renal failure, myocardial infarction, hypertension, peripheral neuropathy, or asthma. Renal involvement occurs in 80% of patients and usually presents the most serious problem; renal failure is the most common cause of death and may follow a rapid or insidious progression of disease.

Most ocular tissues may be similarly affected. The disease most commonly affects the retinal and choroidal circulation, either as a direct result of the vasculitis or indirectly secondary to hypertension; areas of retinal or choroidal ischemia may be revealed by fluorescein angiography.

Scleritis is relatively unusual but, when it occurs, it has a very similar appearance to that seen in WG except that there is very little granuloma formation but much more vascular shutdown. As in WG, any limbal destructive lesions transgress the limbus, but leakage from the capillaries is much less obvious.

Definitive pathological findings are most likely to be provided by renal biopsy, although this is potentially hazardous because of the danger of aneurysm rupture or production of arteriovenous fistulas. A typical lesion demonstrates fibrinoid necrosis of the media of small and medium-sized arteries, particularly at vessel bifurcations, with a pleomorphic cellular infiltrate, predominantly of polymorphonuclear leukocytes with variable numbers of lymphocytes and eosinophils. The normal architecture of the vessel wall is disrupted, and there may be thrombosis or aneurysmal dilatation [44]. Healing with fibrosis may also cause vessel occlusion. Unlike WG, necrotizing granulomas are not a feature. Limited ocular material has been available for examination, but granulomatous and vascular changes have been found in the conjunctiva.

Although immune complexes appear to be the major underlying pathological process, the cause of PAN is not known. Some cases are associated with hepatitis and the presence of hepatitis B antigen, which may form part of the immune complex [45]. This is probably an incidental finding, however, as such complexes are also found in patients with active hepatitis but without vasculitis. Other viruses such as cytomegalovirus, human immunodeficiency virus, and hepatitis A can be associated with a polyarteritis pattern of disease. Although circulating immune complexes can be detected, actual immune complex deposits are found infrequently, suggesting transient deposition or that they are, in fact, not involved in disease pathogenesis [46, 47].

ANCA and, more recently, AECA have been detected in patients with microscopic polyarteritis, a form of PAN limited to involvement of small vessels with associated segmental glomerulonephritis [43, 48]. The reactivity of the latter against endothelial cells suggests their possible involvement in in vivo pathological processes affecting vascular structures in small vessels in primary vasculitides.

Relapsing Polychondritis

Relapsing polychondritis is a rare episodic disorder in which recurrent inflammation occurs in cartilage and other tissues with high concentrations of glycosaminoglycans. The auricular and nasal cartilages are most commonly affected, the latter resulting in painful floppy ears and the loss of the tip of the nose. Tracheal collapse and respiratory obstruction may occur secondary to involvement of the laryngotracheal cartilage. Conductive or sensorineural hearing loss and vestibular dysfunction can result from eustachian tube disease and subsequent serous otitis media and internal auditory artery vasculitis. There is often a fever and a seronegative polyarthritis and, less commonly but associated with a poor prognosis, a systemic vasculitis that may affect any size vessel. Multiple neurological abnormalities have been described and are consistent with vasculitis of the central and peripheral nervous systems. Aneurysm formation and valvular heart disease are also reported. The disease occurs most frequently in middle age and affects individuals of either sex equally. A significant number have an associated autoimmune disorder, typically rheumatoid arthritis.

Ocular complications occur in more than 50% of patients [49]. The most common problems are episcleritis and scleritis, but corneal thinning and melting, uveitis, retinal vasculitis, exudative retinal detachment, optic neuritis, and proptosis with extraocular muscle palsies also occur.

The scleritis is usually anterior and diffuse but, in fact, can be of any type. It is an extremely intractable condition. Of all the patients with scleral disease, these are the most difficult to treat because, although the inflammation rarely causes destruction of the globe or loss of vision, the pain and discomfort are of disabling severity and are very resistant to therapy. It is critical, therefore, to recognize this from the start so that the clinician can support the patient through what is bound to be a prolonged and difficult period.

Histopathological examination of affected cartilage demonstrates a marked perichondritis, decreased basophilia of the matrix representing loss of proteoglycan, and a cellular infiltrate of lymphocytes, histiocytes, plasma cells, and neutrophils [50, 51]. Examination of sclera has revealed a vasculitis thereby confirming that, as in other vasculitides such as WG, rheumatoid arthritis, and PAN, the development of scleritis is a reliable sign of a systemic vasculitis [52].

The cause of relapsing polychondritis is unknown, though it has been considered to be an autoimmune disease due to its association with other autoimmune disorders. Autoantibodies to type II collagen have been detected in relapsing polychondritis, the titers correlating with the severity of disease [53, 54]. As type II collagen is present in both sclera and cartilage, the frequent occurrence of scleritis is not surprising. The presence of a vasculitis suggests the involvement of immune complexes; circulating immune complexes have been detected in some patients, and immunofluorescence studies have demonstrated deposition of immunoglobulin and complement in the vessel walls.

Seronegative Spondyloarthropathies

The seronegative spondyloarthropathies comprise a group of conditions, including ankylosing spondylitis, psoriatic arthritis, Reiter's disease, ulcerative colitis, and Crohn's disease, that have a number of similar features suggesting a common pathogenesis: radiological evidence of sacroileitis, inflammatory peripheral arthritis, absence of serum rheumatoid factor, a familial tendency, and evidence of clinical overlap between members of the group. The majority of ocular manifestations of this group of disorders involve the uveal tract; corneal and scleral disease is uncommon and rarely severe.

The spondyloarthropathies have a strong association with certain HLA types. HLA-B27 is found in more than 90% of cases of ankylosing spondylitis and 75% of cases of Reiter's disease; the prevalence in the general population is 4 to 8% [55–57]. It appears to be a strong marker for the development of anterior uveitis. There is a weaker affinity of HLA-B27 with psoriatic arthritis, ulcerative colitis, and Crohn's disease, but all conditions demonstrate an association of HLA-B27 with a polyarthritis, particularly if spinal involvement is present.

The etiology of these conditions is not known. However, a reactive arthritis may follow certain bowel infections: Reiter's disease has occurred following infection with bacteria such as *Yersinia, Shigella,* and *Salmonella,* while an increased incidence of fecal isolates of *Klebsiella pneumoniae* has been detected in patients with ankylosing spondylitis [58–64]. In these cases, the presence of HLA-B27 is a strong indicator for the development of arthritis. The development of such systemic problems following localized infection may be due to cross-reactivity between bacterial epitopes and HLA-B27 itself [65].

■ Management of Scleral Disease Associated with Systemic Disease

Scleritis in association with systemic disease is generally a manifestation of a systemic vasculitis complicating that disease. As a consequence, it must be taken seriously, and the management of the patient must be undertaken with a physician knowledgeable in the connective tissue disorders.

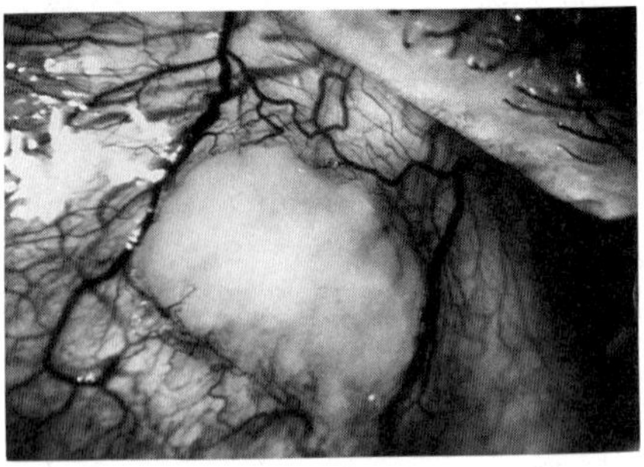

Figure 11 *Treatment with "pulsed" steroid. This 48-year-old patient with necrotizing scleritis accompanying systemic lupus erythematosus (an unusual event) was treated initially with nonsteroidal antiinflammatory agents and then with systemic prednisolone, without improvement. She was then treated with pulsed methylprednisolone and cyclophosphamide, which provided immediate relief of the pain and the lesion started to heal.*

Treatment of scleritis is the systemic treatment of the underlying disease; local therapy plays little or no part. The milder forms of disease may well respond to the nonsteroidal antiinflammatory agents, although not all are equally effective. In general, what has been found to help an individual patient control his or her systemic disease will be effective in controlling his or her scleritis, although the dose may have to be increased. Flurbiprofen, 100 mg three times daily, is usually the most beneficial of the nonsteroidal drugs in the treatment of scleritis.

In necrotizing and severe nonnecrotizing disease, it is necessary to give an immunosuppressive dosage of corticosteroids and, in some cases, such as in Wegener's granulomatosis, further immunosuppressive drugs. Depending on the severity of the condition, steroids can be given orally at a dose of approximately 80 mg prednisolone daily, reducing rapidly to a dosage of 15 mg or less over a period of 2 weeks. In the very acute and severe cases, 1 gm of intravenous "pulsed" methylprednisolone, given slowly over 1 hour and repeated on 2 or 3 occasions in the following week if necessary, can have dramatic results (Figs 11, 12). Oral therapy at a dose of 15 to 20 mg will usually control the disease thereafter. This is potentially dangerous therapy and should be administered only if essential and under close medical supervision.

The treatment of every patient with scleritis or corneal destructive disease is individual, and everyone will require a modification of these regimens or a combination of various medications. With correct treatment, however, almost all patients can be controlled medically, and very few will need additional

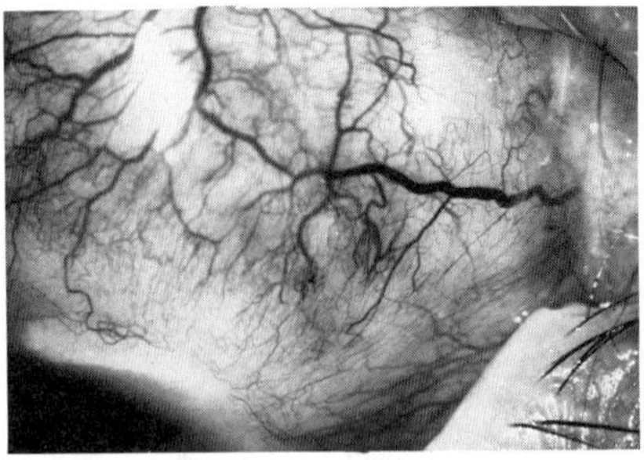

Figure 12 *Appearance of the patient in Figure 11, 1 month later. She was maintained for 6 months on 12.5 mg prednisolone and 100 mg cyclophosphamide per day. The cyclophosphamide was then stopped, and the steroid was eventually withdrawn completely.*

surgery or lose any significant amount of vision. The management of cases of scleritis, although difficult to treat, is rewarding for both doctor and patient.

■ References

1. Watson PG, Hazleman BL. The sclera and systemic disorders. London: Saunders, 1976:45–55
2. Watson PG, Hayreh SS. Scleritis and episcleritis. Br J Ophthalmol 1976;60:163–191
3. Meyer PAR. Patterns of blood flow in episcleral vessels studied by low-dose fluorescein videoangiography. Eye 1988;2:533–546
4. Meyer PAR. The circulation of the human limbus. Eye 1989;3:121–127
5. Watson PG. The nature and the treatment of scleral inflammation. Trans Ophthalmol Soc UK 1982;102:257–281
6. Benson WE. Posterior scleritis. Surv Ophthalmol 1988;32:297–316
7. Calthorpe CM, Watson PG, McCartney ACE. Posterior scleritis: a clinical and histological survey. Eye 1988;2:267–277
8. Sevel D. Necrogranulomatous scleritis. Clinical and histologic features. Am J Ophthalmol 1967;64:1125–1134
9. Young RD, Watson PG. Microscopical studies of necrotising scleritis: I. Cellular aspects. Br J Ophthalmol 1984;68:770–780
10. Watson PG, Young RD. Changes at the periphery of a lesion in necrotising scleritis: anterior segment fluorescein angiography correlated with electron microscopy. Br J Ophthalmol 1985;69:656–663
11. Brawman-Mintzer O, Mondino BJ, Mayer FJ. Distribution of complement in the sclera. Invest Ophthalmol Vis Sci 1989;30:2240–2244
12. Rao NA, Marak GE, Hidayat AA. Necrotizing scleritis. A clinico-pathologic study of 41 cases. Ophthalmology 1985;92:1542–1549
13. McGavin DDM, Williamson J, Forrester JV, et al. Episcleritis and scleritis. A study of their clinical manifestations and association with rheumatoid arthritis. Br J Ophthalmol 1976;60:192–226
14. Lyne AJ. "Contact lens" cornea in rheumatoid arthritis. Br J Ophthalmol 1970; 54:410–415
15. Bankhurst AD, Husby G, Williams RC. Predominance of T-cells in the lymphocytic infiltrates of synovial tissue in rheumatoid arthritis. Arthritis Rheum 1976;19: 555–562
16. Moore K, Walters MT, Jones DB, et al. An immunohistological study of CD4+ lymphocyte subsets within inflammatory lesions with special reference to rheumatoid arthritis and inflammatory bowel disease. Immunology 1988;65:457–463
17. Doita M, Maeda S, Kawai K, et al. Analysis of lymphocyte subsets of bone marrow in patients with rheumatoid arthritis by two colour immunofluorescence and flow cytometry. Ann Rheum Dis 1990;49:168–171
18. Carpenter AB, Eisenbeis CH Jr, Carrabis S, et al. Soluble interleukin-2 receptor: elevated levels in serum and synovial fluid of patients with rheumatoid arthritis. J Clin Lab Anal 1990;4:130–134
19. Stastny P, Ball EJ, Khan MA, et al. HLA-DR4 and other genetic markers in rheumatoid arthritis. Br J Rheumatol 1988;27[suppl 2](1):132–138
20. McMichael AJ, Sasazuki T, McDevitt HO, Payne RO. Increased frequency of HLA-Cw3 and HLA-Dw4 in rheumatoid arthritis. Arthritis Rheum 1977;20:1037–1042
21. Cassidy JT, Levinson JE, Bass JC, et al. A study of classification criteria for a diagnosis of juvenile rheumatoid arthritis. Arthritis Rheum 1986;29:274–281
22. Kanski JJ. Juvenile arthritis and uveitis. Surv Ophthalmol 1990;34:253–267
23. Hargraves MM, Richmond H, Morton R. Presentation of two bone marrow elements: the "tart" cell and the "LE" cell. Proc Mayo Clin 1948;23:25–28

24. Morrow WJW, Isenberg DA. Auto-immune rheumatic diseases. Oxford: Blackwell Scientific, 1987
25. Asherson RA, Merry P, Acheson JF, et al. Antiphospholipid antibodies: a risk factor for occlusive vascular disease in systemic lupus erythematosus and the "primary" antiphospholipid syndrome. Ann Rheum Dis 1989;48:358–361
26. Aronson AJ, Ordonez NG, Diddie KR, Ernest TJ. Immune-complex deposition in the eye in systemic lupus erythematosus. Arch Intern Med 1979;139:1312–1313
27. Karpik AG, Schwartz MM, Dickey LE, et al. Ocular immune reactants in patients dying with systemic lupus erythematosus. Clin Immunol Immunopathol 1985; 35:295–312
28. Schoenfeld Y, Isenberg D. DNA antibody idiotype: a review of their genetic, clinical, and immunopathologic features. Semin Arthritis Rheum 1987;16:245–252
29. Schoenfeld Y, Vilner Y, Reshef T, et al. Increased presence of common systemic lupus erythematosus (SLE) anti-DNA idiotypes (16/6 Id, 32/15 Id) is induced by procainamide. J Clin Immunol 1987;7:410–419
30. Froelich CJ, Guiffant S, Sosenko M, Muth K. Deficient interleukin-2-activated killer cell cytotoxicity in patients with systemic lupus erythematosus. Clin Immunol Immunopathol 1989;50:132–145
31. Hishikawa T, Tokano Y, Sekigawa I, et al. HLA-DP+ T cells and deficient interleukin-2 production in patients with systemic lupus erythematosus. Clin Immunol Immunopathol 1990;55:285–296
32. Godman GC, Churg J. Wegener's granulomatosis. Pathology and review of the literature. Arch Pathol 1954;58:533–553
33. Haynes BF, Fishman ML, Fauci AS, Wolff SM. The ocular manifestations of Wegener's granulomatosis. Fifteen years' experience and review of the literature. Am J Med 1977;63:131–141
34. Bullen CL, Liesegang TJ, McDonald TJ, DeRemee RA. Ocular complications of Wegener's granulomatosis. Ophthalmology 1983;90:279–290
35. Feinberg R. Necrotizing granulomatosis and angiitis of the lungs with massive splenic necrosis and focal thrombotic granulomatous glomerulonephritis. Am J Clin Pathol 1953;23:413–428
36. Devaney KO, Travis WD, Hoffman G, et al. Interpretation of head and neck biopsies in Wegener's granulomatosis. A pathological study of 126 biopsies in 70 patients. Am J Surg Pathol 1990;14:555–564
37. Pinching AJ, Rees AJ, Pussell BA, et al. Relapses in Wegener's granulomatosis: the role of infection. Br Med J 1980;281:836–838
38. Van der Woude FJ, Rasmussen N, Lobatto S, et al. Autoantibodies against neutrophils and monocytes: tool for diagnosis and marker of disease activity in Wegener's granulomatosis. Lancet 1985;1:425–429
39. Savige JA, Gallichio M, Georgiou T, Davies DJ. Diverse target antigens recognised by circulating antibodies in anti-neutrophil cytoplasm antibody-associated renal vasculitides. Clin Exp Immunol 1990;82:238–243
40. Falk RJ, Jenette JC. Anti-neutrophil cytoplasm antibodies with specificity for myeloperoxidase in patients with systemic vasculitis and idiopathic necrotising and crescentic glomerulonephritis. N Engl J Med 1988;318:1651–1657
41. Ludemann J, Utecht B, Gross WL. Anti-neutrophil cytoplasm antibodies in Wegener's granulomatosis recognise an elastinolytic enzyme. J Exp Med 1990;171: 357–362
42. Jenette JC, Wilkman AS, Falk RJ. Anti-neutrophil cytoplasmic autoantibody-associated glomerulonephritis and vasculitis. Am J Pathol 1989;135:921–930
43. Ferraro G, Meroni PL, Tincani A, et al. Anti-endothelial cell antibodies in patients with Wegener's granulomatosis and micropolyarteritis. Clin Exp Immunol 1990; 79:47–53
44. D'Agati V, Chander P, Nash M, Mancilla-Jimenez R. Idiopathic microscopic polyar-

teritis nodosa: ultrastructural observations on the renal and vascular and glomerular lesions. Am J Kidney Dis 1986;7:95–110
45. Michalak T. Immune complexes of hepatitis B surface antigen in the pathogenesis of periarteritis nodosa. A study of seven necropsy cases. Am J Pathol 1978;90: 619–632
46. Ronco P, Verroust P, Mignon F, et al. Immunopathological studies of polyarteritis nodosa and Wegener's granulomatosis: a report of 43 patients with 51 renal biopsies. Q J Med 1983;206:213–226
47. Barratt J, Sindrey M, Summerly R, et al. Circulating immune complexes in cutaneous and systemic vasculitis: clinicopathological correlations. Ann Rheum Dis 1982; 41:25–29
48. Savage CO, Lockwood CM. Autoantibodies in primary systemic vasculitis. Adv Intern Med 1990:35:73–92
49. Isaak BL, Liesegang TJ, Michet CJ. Ocular and systemic findings in relapsing polychondritis. Ophthalmology 1986;93:681–689
50. Giroux L, Paquin F, Guerard-Desjardins MJ, Lefaivre A. Relapsing polychondritis: an autoimmune disease. Semin Arthritis Rheum 1983;13:182–187
51. Valanzuela R, Cooperrider PA, Gogate P, et al. Relapsing polychondritis. Immunomicroscopic findings in cartilage of ear biopsy specimens. Hum Pathol 1980; 11:19–22
52. Hoang-Xuan T, Foster CS, Rice BA. Scleritis in relapsing polychondritis. Response to therapy. Ophthalmology 1990;97:892–898
53. Foidart JM, Abe S, Martin GR, et al. Antibodies to type II collagen in relapsing polychondritis. N Engl J Med 1978;299:1203–1207
54. Ebringer R, Rook G, Swana GT, et al. Autoantibodies to cartilage and type II collagen in relapsing polychondritis and other rheumatic disease. Ann Rheum Dis 1981;40:473–479
55. Brewerton DA, Caffrey M, Hart FD, et al. Ankylosing spondylitis and HL-A27. Lancet 1973;1:904–907
56. Brewerton DA, Caffrey M, Nicholls A, et al. Acute anterior uveitis and HL-A27. Lancet 1973;2:994–996
57. Brewerton DA, Caffrey M, Nicholls A, et al. Reiter's disease and HL-A27. Lancet 1973;2:996–998
58. Ebringer RW, Cawdell DR, Cowling P, Ebringer A. Sequential studies in ankylosing spondylitis: association of *Klebsiella pneumoniae* with active disease. Ann Rheum Dis 1978;37:146–151
59. Ebringer A, Cox NL, Abuljadayel I, et al. *Klebsiella* antibodies in ankylosing spondylitis and *Proteus* antibodies in rheumatoid arthritis. Br J Rheumatol 1988;27(suppl 2):72–85
60. Paronen I. Reiter's disease, a study of 344 cases observed in Finland. Acta Med Scand 1948;131(suppl 213):1–114
61. Amor B. Chlamydia and Reiter's syndrome. Br J Rheumatol 1983;22(suppl 2): 156–160
62. Solem JH, Lassen J. Reiter's disease following *Yersinia enterocolitica* infection. Scand J Infect Dis 1971;3:83–85
63. Leirisalo-Repo M, Skylv G, Kousa M. Follow-up study of Reiter's disease and reactive arthritis. Factors influencing the natural course and prognosis. Clin Rheumatol 1987;6(suppl 2):73–82
64. Warren CPW. Arthritis associated with *Salmonella* infection. Ann Rheum Dis 1970;29:483–487
65. Husby G, Tsuchiya N, Schwimmbeck PL, et al. Cross-reactive epitope with *Klebsiella pneumoniae* nitrogenase in articular tissue of HLA B27 positive patients with ankylosing spondylitis. Arthritis Rheum 1989;32:437–445

Systemic Associations of Anterior Uveitis

James T. Rosenbaum, M.D.

A recent study reported that 50% of patients with anterior uveitis have a causally related systemic illness such as Reiter's syndrome, ankylosing spondylitis, juvenile rheumatoid arthritis, inflammatory bowel disease, or interstitial nephritis (Table 1) [1]. This chapter reviews the clinical features and pathophysiology of the diseases associated with anterior uveitis. In many instances, the attributes of the uveitis are sufficiently distinctive that the diagnosis of the systemic illness is first suspected by the ocular presentation.

Spondyloarthropathy

Reiter's syndrome and ankylosing spondylitis are both forms of spondyloarthropathy (Table 2). Each has a strong association with the histocompatibility marker known as HLA-B27. Approximately 20% of patients with either Reiter's syndrome or ankylosing spondylitis will develop a characteristic anterior uveitis. Reiter's syndrome was described by the German physician, Hans Reiter. Classically, it is a reactive arthritis that begins subsequent to a nongonococcal urethritis or diarrhea secondary to *Salmonella, Shigella, Yersinia,* or *Campylobacter* infection. Common manifestations of Reiter's syndrome include arthritis, conjunctivitis, and nongonococcal urethritis. The arthritis is typically asymmetrical and especially involves the sacroiliac joints as well as the joints of the lower extremities. Digits may develop a characteristic sausage swelling known as *dactylitis.* Tendons including the Achilles and the plantar fascia are commonly involved. Skin and mucosal involvement may include shallow oral aphthae or a psoriaform rash on the palms, soles, or the glans penis. Sixty to ninety percent of patients with Reiter's syndrome possess the HLA-B27 antigen; this compares to 6 to 8% of the white population in the United States.

Ankylosing spondylitis is closely related to Reiter's syndrome. Ninety percent of patients with ankylosing spondylitis are HLA-B27-positive. The *sine qua non* of ankylosing spondylitis is the development of bilateral sacroiliitis [2]. Typically, this results in low back pain that begins insidiously, is associated with morning stiffness, improves with exercise, and does not cause radiation of pain along a dermatomal pattern [3]. The majority of patients with either Reiter's

Table 1 *Systemic Diseases Associated with Iritis*

Acute leukemia
Adenoviral infection
Ankylosing spondylitis
Anterior segment ischemia
Behçet's disease
Crohn's disease
Drug or hypersensitivity reaction
Interstitial nephritis
Juvenile rheumatoid arthritis
Kawasaki disease
Leprosy
Leptospirosis
Lyme disease
Multiple sclerosis
Mumps
Psoriatic arthritis
Reiter's syndrome
Relapsing polychondritis
Sarcoidosis
Sjögren's syndrome
Syphilis
Systemic lupus erythematosus
Tuberculosis
Ulcerative colitis
Vogt-Koyanagi-Harada syndrome
Wegener's granulomatosis

syndrome or ankylosing spondylitis are male. Patients with ankylosing spondylitis frequently develop a peripheral arthritis identical to that seen in Reiter's syndrome. As is true for Reiter's syndrome, roughly 20% of patients with ankylosing spondylitis will develop an anterior uveitis.

Characteristic Features of Associated Uveitis

The uveitis associated with either of these HLA-B27-associated diseases is highly characteristic (Table 3) [4, 5]. In virtually all patients, the initial episode begins acutely and unilaterally. Pain and redness are prominent features. A 1- to 2-day prodrome may precede the actual appearance of cell and flare in the anterior chamber. The uveitis is more common in men than women. Intraocular pressure usually is lowered by an acute episode; posterior synechiae commonly form; and cystoid macular edema is a more frequent complication than with other forms of anterior uveitis. A plastic iritis or hypopyon can also be seen with this disease. Despite the frequent fulminant nature of the inflammation, the visual prognosis is good. The episode usually resolves within 2 to 4 months with a return to normal acuity. However, the episodes are frequently recurrent. Chorioretinal involvement does not occur, but a marked cellular reaction in the vitreous is present in a minority of patients.

Table 2 *Comparative Features of Reiter's Syndrome and Ankylosing Spondylitis*

Feature	Reiter's Syndrome	Ankylosing Spondylitis
Sacroiliitis	Usual	Always
Peripheral arthritis	Usual	Common
HLA-B27-associated	60–90%	90%
Acute anterior uveitis	20%	20%
Nongonococcal urethritis	Usual	Not associated
Conjunctivitis	Often	Not associated
Aphthous stomatitis	Occasional	Not associated
Psoriaform rash	Occasional	Not associated
Nail changes	Occasional	Not associated
Precipitated by urethral or intestinal infection	Often	No
Predominant in men	Yes	Yes

Of all patients with anterior uveitis, approximately 50% are HLA-B27-positive [6]. If one considers the subset of anterior uveitis that is unilateral, has an acute onset, and is not secondary to a known other cause such as herpes simplex or surgical trauma, a far higher percentage will be HLA-B27-associated [4]. The majority of patients with HLA-B27-associated iritis will have accompanying arthritis involving the back, peripheral joints, or both [4, 7]. Reiter's syndrome and ankylosing spondylitis are easily the most common systemic illnesses associated with uveitis in the United States, accounting for 13% of all uveitis diagnoses and 25% of all anterior uveitis diagnoses in one recent report from a uveitis survey clinic [1]. HLA-B27 is also associated with a subset of patients who develop psoriatic arthritis and with children who develop juvenile ankylosing spondylitis, which is frequently included as a subset of juvenile rheumatoid arthritis (see page 136) [8]. Patients with either psoriatic arthritis or juvenile ankylosing spondylitis may develop a unilateral, acute-onset anterior uveitis as is seen with other HLA-B27-associated diseases. In fact, these diseases and others associated with inflammation in the sacroiliac

Table 3 *Hallmarks of HLA-B27-Associated Uveitis*

Acute in onset
Unilateral
Anterior
Often recurrent
Usually in males
Usually associated with joint disease
Short duration (<4 months)
Often associated with synechiae and cystoid macular edema
Rarely associated with glaucoma
Occasionally associated with fibrin or hypopyon

Table 4 *Causes of Sacroiliitis Associated with Iritis*

Ankylosing spondylitis
Reiter's syndrome
Crohn's disease
Ulcerative colitis
Psoriatic arthritis
Behçet's disease

joints have in common involvement of the anterior uveal tract as a feature (Table 4).

Stuuies of the Pathogenesis of HLA-B27-Associated Diseases

The cause of HLA-B27-associated diseases is being studied intensively. At least six subtypes of HLA-B27 have been recognized [9], but each subtype appears to predispose equally to inflammatory joint disease. The HLA-B27 gene has been cloned and the structure of the B27 peptide analyzed. Various investigators have reported cross-reactivities between HLA-B27 and several gram-negative bacteria [10]. A six–amino acid stretch of HLA-B27 appears to be identical to amino acids in an enzyme produced by *Klebsiella,* and it has been proposed that this molecular mimicry would result in the production of autoantibodies [11]. Two animal models [12], adjuvant arthritis and endotoxin-induced uveitis [13], may be relevant to understanding the spondyloarthropathies. Some strains of rats will develop a reactive arthritis after a footpad injection of killed mycobacteria. The arthritis involves the spine and sacroiliac joints much like Reiter's syndrome or ankylosing spondylitis. Furthermore, the footpad injection results in nonarticular disease including uveitis and nongonococcal urethritis. Unlike the human disease, the uveitis may be granulomatous. Intriguingly, the T lymphocytes that appear to cause this disease may be responding to a specific heat shock protein.

Endotoxin-induced uveitis results from the footpad, intravenous, or intraperitoneal injection of endotoxin into laboratory animals such as rats or rabbits. The dose of endotoxin that induces anterior uveitis does not cause light-microscopical changes in other organs. This model's potential relevance is enhanced by the reported cross-reactions between HLA-B27 and gram-negative bacteria, the ability of gram-negative infections to trigger Reiter's syndrome, and the similar eye, joint, and skin manifestations shared by inflammatory bowel disease and Reiter's syndrome. Due to bowel inflammation, endotoxemia may occur with active inflammatory bowel disease [14]. Occult bowel inflammation that can be detected by colonoscopy and which is histologically similar to Crohn's disease has been detected in the majority of patients with either Reiter's syndrome or ankylosing spondylitis [15]. Endotoxin-induced uveitis differs from Reiter's syndrome–associated uveitis by virtue of its bilaterality and its lack of association with a major histocompatibility complex allele.

Perhaps the biggest breakthrough in the understanding of Reiter's syndrome and ankylosing spondylitis may come from the creation of HLA-B27-positive transgenic rodents. In one recent report, rats that express the human HLA-B27 gene appear to develop a spontaneous arthritis [16]. Possible eye pathology in this model has been described. The pathogenesis of this disease will undoubtedly relate to Reiter's syndrome and ankylosing spondylitis.

■ Sarcoidosis

Ocular disease is frequently the initial manifestation of sarcoidosis [17]. Conversely, sarcoidosis is the second most common systemic illness associated with uveitis, as reported in a recent review from a United States referral clinic [1]. The cause of sarcoidosis is unknown. Histologically, the disease is characterized by noncaseating granulomas. This pathological response is most typically present in the lung and mediastinal lymph nodes. Similar abnormal findings, however, can sometimes be found in such diverse organs as skin, joint, liver, oral mucosa, heart, and central nervous system. Symptoms of sarcoidosis vary widely depending on the distribution of pathology. Many patients with sarcoidosis are asymptomatic. The ocular manifestations are protean and include a dry eye, conjunctival or eyelid involvement, orbital pseudotumor, scleritis, band keratopathy, and optic neuritis. Uveal involvement can take many forms including an acute-onset iritis, retinal vasculitis, insidious-onset anterior or posterior involvement, chorioretinitis, or a combination of these [17, 18]. Although iritis alone is not the typical presentation of ocular sarcoidosis, this diagnosis may be the initial manifestation of the disease. The diagnosis of sarcoidosis should always be considered in any patient presenting with an iritis of unknown etiology.

The diagnosis of sarcoidosis is most reliably established by a biopsy that demonstrates the typical pathology and then the exclusion of other causes of granulomatous inflammation such as fungal or mycobacterial infection. Possible biopsy sites include lymph nodes, lung, skin, oral mucosa, and conjunctiva. Patients with sarcoidosis commonly have a variety of laboratory abnormalities, including elevated serum angiotensin-converting enzyme and lysozyme levels as well as anergic responses to skin test antigens. The laboratory findings are not sufficiently unique to establish a diagnosis. However, the combination of uveitis and *symmetrical* hilar adenopathy is sufficiently specific for sarcoidosis that our practice has not been to obtain tissue confirmation when this presentation occurs [19], and noninvasive tests such as the angiotensin-converting enzyme level support the diagnosis.

The prognosis for ocular sarcoidosis is variable. A Finnish study indicates that many patients will have inactive pulmonary disease within 3 years from onset [18], but the eye problems may be more persistent. If the ocular inflammation is bilateral, not controlled by topical medications, and severe enough to alter daily activities, oral corticosteroids are indicated. In many patients, corticosteroids are dramatically effective and can usually be tapered to an alternate-day schedule with maintenance of acceptable acuity. The goal for therapy should not necessarily be elimination of disease activity. The treating physician should balance the benefit of the medication with concern for toxicity. Accordingly, a dosing schedule might be chosen that makes a compromise between benefit and risk.

■ Juvenile Rheumatoid Arthritis

The term *juvenile rheumatoid arthritis* (JRA) is misleading. JRA can be subdivided into several distinct subsets, four of which are indicated in Table 5. Only 10% of children with JRA have a disease that mimics rheumatoid arthritis in adults. Like adults with rheumatoid arthritis, these children commonly develop a dry eye (secondary Sjögren's syndrome) and occasionally develop scleritis. They are not at increased risk for iritis except for the anterior chamber inflammation that may be secondary to scleritis. Some children with a diagnosis of JRA are HLA-B27-positive, have an arthritis similar in type and distribution to adults with either Reiter's syndrome or ankylosing spondylitis and, like their adult counterparts, have roughly a 20% likelihood of developing an acute-onset, unilateral iritis. Some children labeled as having JRA have an illness that has also been termed *Still's disease.* This diagnosis should be reserved for children (and occasionally adults) who have a disease characterized by fever, an evanescent rash, hepatosplenomegaly, adenopathy, leukocytosis, and arthritis. These children are at low risk for the development of iritis [20].

Approximately 20% of children with JRA fall into the subset that is strongly associated with the development of iritis [21, 22]. These children are usually female, their disease generally begins between the ages of 4 and 8, their antinuclear antibody test is usually positive but rheumatoid factor is not detectable, and commonly only a few joints are involved. Roughly 50% of children in this subset will develop a highly characteristic anterior uveitis. The eye disease may precede the joint disease, develop subsequent to it, or present as a forme fruste of the disease without clinically significant joint disease. The eye disease is usually bilateral and insidious in onset; the duration is usually chronic. Children with this form of iridocyclitis frequently develop all the possible complications of ocular inflammation including band keratopathy, cataract, glaucoma, posterior synechiae, and cystoid macular edema. The activity of the eye inflammation does not correlate well with the pace of the joint

Table 5 *Characteristic Features of Subsets of Juvenile Rheumatoid Arthritis (JRA)*

Distinguishing Features of Subsets of JRA	Iritis
Polyarticular, symmetrical joint disease, positive rheumatoid factor, usually affects girls	Not associated
Systemic onset, fever, evanescent rash, hepatosplenomegaly (Still's disease)	Rare
Pauciarticular, positive antinuclear antibodies, usually affects girls, onset before age 9	Frequent bilateral insidious-onset iritis
Pauciarticular, no autoantibodies, HLA-B27-positive, usually affects boys	Unilateral, acute-onset iritis

disease. Patients within this subset should be followed carefully for the development of this ocular complication. If iridocyclitis does develop, the treating ophthalmologist needs to follow the course of the disease closely, since flares can be accompanied by minimal symptoms. The goal of topical therapy should be to minimize but not eliminate the inflammation, since chronically administered aggressive topical therapy will eventually result in complications such as cataractogenesis.

■ Inflammatory Bowel Disease

Both forms of inflammatory bowel disease—Crohn's disease and ulcerative colitis—can be associated with iritis as well as other ocular manifestations such as episcleritis and scleritis [23, 24]. In general, the iritis associated with inflammatory bowel disease is similar to that seen with the HLA-B27 spectrum of joint diseases. Typically, the iritis is acute in onset, unilateral, and self-limited. It is more likely to occur with active bowel disease. The likelihood of eye inflammation correlates well with the presence of other extraintestinal manifestations of the disease such as arthritis, rash, and aphthous stomatitis. Crohn's disease, like sarcoidosis, is a granulomatous process. Although Crohn's disease will usually be associated with a unilateral iritis, like sarcoidosis it may result in intraocular inflammation that is bilateral, posterior, chronic, or associated with a retinal vasculitis.

■ Behçet's Disease

Behçet's disease is diagnosed by the triad of aphthous stomatitis, genital ulceration, and uveitis [25]. Ocular disease occurs in approximately 80% of patients with Behçet's. Other manifestations include arthritis, diarrhea, erythema nodosum, and sterile meningitis. The disease has strong ethnic relationships. In Japan, it is the most common cause of uveitis. It is also common in middle Eastern countries. It is associated with the HLA antigen, B51.

Behçet's disease often causes a bilateral iritis. More posterior inflammation and a retinal vasculitis are also characteristic. All aspects of Behçet's disease are usually episodic, with a tendency to remit and exacerbate spontaneously. Treatment of this condition has been frustrating with generally inadequate responses to oral or topical corticosteroids. Recent reports have indicated very promising results with either cyclosporine A [26] or azathioprine [27]. Neither agent should be considered a cure, but both seem to result in fewer and less severe disease flares.

■ Interstitial Nephritis

Interstitial nephritis is a rare disease characterized by azotemia and leukocytes in the urine. Interstitial nephritis may be idiopathic or it may be triggered by a presumed allergic reaction to medications such as antibiotics or nonsteroidal antiinflammatory drugs. The disease is more common in children than adults. Despite the rarity of interstitial nephritis, it ranks as one of the more common systemic illnesses found in association with iritis [1, 28]. The eye disease is quite characteristic. It is usually bilateral, although it may be asymmetrical in its intensity and may begin unilaterally. The onset is usually acute, with a moderate degree of eye pain and redness. The eye disease is generally confined to the anterior segment. Patients with this form of iritis will often have systemic complaints such as fever, fatigue, anorexia, or abdominal pain. They may have anemia and mildly abnormal liver function tests. The recognition of this distinct entity is critical for a number of reasons. The renal disease may progress to renal failure if untreated. The disease may respond to an intervention as simple as discontinuing an over-the-counter nonsteroidal anti-inflammatory drug and, if necessary, the disease usually responds promptly to oral corticosteroids.

■ Sjögren's Syndrome

Sjögren's syndrome refers to the combination of dry eyes and dry mouth resulting from an apparent autoimmune inflammation. Recent interest has focused on Epstein-Barr virus or a retrovirus as a possible cause for this condition [29]. Sjögren's syndrome can be diagnosed by objective evidence for dry eyes and dry mouth as well as the detection of autoantibodies including antinuclear antibodies, rheumatoid factor, and antibodies to Sjögren's syndrome antigen A and B (SS-A and SS-B, respectively). A minor salivary gland biopsy should reveal a lymphocytic infiltrate. Sjögren's syndrome may be secondary to another connective tissue disease such as rheumatoid arthritis or systemic lupus erythematosus, or it may be primary (i.e., unassociated with a recognizable connective tissue syndrome). In either case, Sjögren's may affect other exocrine glands with resultant dryness of respiratory secretions, skin, and vagina. Frequent systemic manifestations include arthritis, neuropathy, vasculitis, interstitial pneumonia, lymphadenopathy, fatigue, and depression. Laboratory findings include the autoantibodies previously mentioned, an elevated erythrocyte sedimentation rate, increased gamma globulins, and mild anemia.

Sjögren's syndrome does not ordinarily result in intraocular inflammation. However, a group of predominantly female patients with dry eyes, positive tests for antinuclear antibodies, elevated sedimentation rates, systemic complaints such as fatigue and arthralgias, and abnormal minor salivary gland biopsies has been reported to develop a chronic iritis in association with cells in the vitreous humor [30]. Granulomatous keratic precipitates, synechiae, cataract, and increased intraocular pressure may complicate this chronic form of intraocular inflammation.

■ Vogt-Koyanagi-Harada Syndrome

Vogt-Koyanagi-Harada syndrome is an autoimmune form of uveitis [31]. The complete spectrum of the disease includes a sterile meningitis, alopecia, vitiligo, poliosis (patchy whitening of the eyelash or hair in the scalp), and eighth nerve disease (tinnitus, dizziness, hearing loss, or dysacusis). The disease has a strong ethnic predisposition. It is common in people of Japanese descent. In the United States, it is confined mostly to Mexican Americans and native American Indians. Although the pathogenesis is unknown, one theory is that it represents an autoimmune attack directed against melanin-containing cells. The iritis in this disease is often fulminant. The retinal findings are more distinctive and characteristic. The retinal findings classically include serous retinal detachments, which are found bilaterally.

■ Kawasaki Disease

Kawasaki disease is a form of vasculitis that occurs in childhood [32]. It is also known as the mucocutaneous lymph node syndrome. Some consider it to be a juvenile form of polyarteritis nodosa. Conjunctivitis is a prominent manifestation of this disease. One of its hallmarks is coronary arteritis. A mild bilateral iritis is present in approximately 80% of patients with Kawasaki disease [33], although the iritis is often overlooked because of the severity of the other systemic manifestations. The prognosis for the iritis is excellent, often with mild, self-limited disease.

■ Multiple Sclerosis

Multiple sclerosis is not usually associated with uveitis. Optic neuritis is the most common ocular manifestation of this immunologically mediated neurological disease. An intermediate uveitis is occasionally present in patients with multiple sclerosis [34]. A granulomatous bilateral anterior uveitis is a rare but very distinctive association with multiple sclerosis [35].

■ Miscellaneous Conditions

A variety of viral illnesses commonly are associated with a mild iritis [36]. Adenoviral infections, mumps, and influenza are examples. The iritis is generally limited in duration and without visually significant consequences. The most common viral illnesses that cause clinically significant anterior uveitis are herpes simplex and herpes zoster. However, ordinarily these are not systemic illnesses at the time of active iritis. Leptospirosis, a spirochetal disease with liver and central nervous system manifestations, may cause anterior uveitis. Leprosy can cause anterior segment inflammation [37]. Tuberculosis is a rare cause of anterior uveitis. The diagnosis of tuberculosis should be considered in the case of granulomatous disease, inflammation that is refractory to corticosteroids, uveitis in a debilitated host, or in patients with active pulmonary tuberculosis.

Serum sickness or adverse reactions to medications such as sulfonamides can produce an iritis that is usually bilateral and acute in onset [38]. Although iritis is uncommon as a reaction to medications, it is essential to remember this possibility in the differential diagnosis. Often, other manifestations of drug toxicity will be present as well.

Cells in the anterior chamber may be the initial manifestation of an acute leukemia [39]. This masquerade syndrome should be considered in children presenting with iritis.

Finally, a variety of other systemic illnesses can result in iritis. These illnesses include systemic lupus erythematosus [40], Wegener's granulomatosis [41], syphilis [42], Lyme disease [43], and relapsing polychondritis [44]. Each illness in this group has other ocular manifestations that are more characteristic than iritis. Ischemia of the anterior segment can occasionally masquerade as inflammation and present as eye discomfort with cell and flare in the aqueous humor. Still other systemic illnesses defy diagnostic categorization. The finding of iritis in the setting of an undiagnosed systemic illness should suggest the possibility of an immunologically mediated or infectious disease. The proper evaluation should always include a thorough medical history as well as a chest roentgenogram and a serological test for syphilis.

■ Comments

Despite the multitude of systemic diseases associated with iritis and the significant likelihood that a patient with iritis does have a systemic disease, internists, family practitioners, and other nonophthalmological diagnosticians are generally ignorant about anterior uveitis. Major textbooks of medicine, for example, usually do not include discussions of the differential diagnosis of anterior uveitis. Internists are not generally aware that distinguishing features of the inflammation—such as the precise location, duration, onset, symmetry, and associated ocular complications—can be useful diagnostically. Only an exceptional internist realizes that illnesses such as Reiter's syndrome, ankylosing spondylitis, juvenile rheumatoid arthritis, sarcoidosis, and interstitial nephritis are frequently associated with an iritis, whereas anterior uveitis is a rare manifestation of illnesses such as systemic lupus erythematosus and leptospirosis. This ignorance is illustrated in the proceedings of a recent clinical pathological conference published in a prestigious medical journal [45]: In reporting on a patient with sarcoidosis, the discussant states that iritis "may be caused by sarcoidosis, syphilis, tuberculosis, or rheumatoid arthritis." He omits the diseases most commonly associated with iritis and includes rare associations (syphilis and tuberculosis) and a disease (rheumatoid arthritis) that is not associated with iritis. It is, therefore, essential that ophthalmologists be familiar with the systemic diseases associated with iritis. Seeking medical consultation for patients with iritis is appropriate, but the ophthalmologist may need to educate the consultant as to the systemic illnesses that are most likely to be found based on the ocular disease.

This work was supported in part by Research to Prevent Blindness, Inc., New York, NY, and grant EY-06484 from the National Eye Institute.

■ References

1. Rosenbaum JT. Uveitis. An internist's view. Arch Intern Med 1989;149:1173–1176
2. The HSG, Steven MM, van der Linden SM, Cats A. Evaluation of diagnostic criteria for ankylosing spondylitis. Br J Rheumatol 1985;24:242–249
3. Calin A, Porta J, Fries JF, Schurman DJ. Clinical history as a screening test for ankylosing spondylitis. JAMA 1977;237:2613–2614
4. Rosenbaum JT. Characterization of uveitis associated with spondyloarthritis. J Rheumatol 1989;16:792–796
5. Rothova A, van Veenedaal MS, Linssen A, et al. Clinical features of acute anterior uveitis. Am J Ophthalmol 1987;103:137–145
6. Brewerton DA, Caffrey M, Nicholls A, et al. Acute anterior uveitis and HLA B27. Lancet 1973;2:994–996
7. Feltkamp TEW. HLA B27, acute anterior uveitis, and ankylosing spondylitis. Adv Inflamm Res 1985;9:211–216
8. Sheerin KA, Giannini EH, Brewer EJ, Barron KS. HLA-B27-associated arthropathy in childhood: long-term clinical and diagnostic outcome. Arthritis Rheum 1988; 31:1165–1170
9. Bodmer JG, Marsh SGE, Parham P, et al. Nomenclature for factors of the HLA system, 1989. Hum Immunol 1990;28:326–342
10. Zhang J-J, Hamachi M, Hamachi T, et al. The bacterial outer membrane protein that reacts with anti-HLA-B27 antibodies is the OMPA protein. J Immunol 1989;143:2955–2960
11. Schwimmbeck PL, Oldstone MB. *Klebsiella pneumoniae* and HLA B27-associated diseases of Reiter's syndrome and ankylosing spondylitis. Curr Top Microbiol Immunol 1989;144:45–56
12. Rosenbaum JT. Why HLA-B27: an analysis based on two animal models. Ann Intern Med 1981;94:261–263
13. Rosenbaum JT, McDevitt HO, Guss RB, Egbert PR. Endotoxin-induced uveitis in rats as a model for human disease. Nature 1980;286:611–613
14. Aoki K. A study of endotoxemia in ulcerative colitis and Crohn's disease: I. Clinical study. Acta Med Okayama 1978;32:147–158
15. Mielants H, Erick M, Veys RJ, et al. Repeat ileocolonoscopy in reactive arthritis. J Rheumatol 1987;14:456–458
16. Hammer RE, Maika SD, Richardson JA, et al. Spontaneous inflammatory disease in transgenic rats expressing HLA-B27 and human beta-2 microglobulin: an animal model of HLA-B27-associated human disorders. Cell 1990;63:1099–1112
17. Obenauf CD, Shaw HE, Sydnor CF, Klintworth GK. Sarcoidosis and its ophthalmic manifestations. Am J Ophthalmol 1978;86:648–655
18. Karma A, Huhti E, Poukkula A. Course and outcome of ocular sarcoidosis. Am J Ophthalmol 1988;106:467–472
19. Winterbauer RH, Belic N, Moores KD. A clinical interpretation of bilateral hilar adenopathy. Ann Intern Med 1973;78:65–71
20. Rosenbaum JT. Iridocyclitis is not characteristic of Still's disease. West J Med 1985;143:252
21. Litvin DG, Wallace K, Chylack L, et al. Early-onset pauciarticular juvenile rheumatoid arthritis associated with human leukocyte antigen-DRw5, iritis, and antinuclear antibody. J Clin Invest 1980;66:426–429
22. Schaller JG, Johnson GD, Holborrow EJ, et al. The association of antinuclear antibodies with the chronic iridocyclitis of juvenile rheumatoid arthritis (Still's disease). Arthritis Rheum 1974;17:409–416
23. Korelitz BI, Coles RS. Uveitis (iritis) associated with ulcerative and granulomatous colitis. Gastroenterology 1967;52:78–82

24. Danzi JT. Extraintestinal manifestations of idiopathic inflammatory bowel disease. Arch Intern Med 1988;148:297–302
25. Colvard DM, Robertson DM, O'Duffy JD. The ocular manifestations of Behçet's disease. Arch Ophthalmol 1977;95:1813–1817
26. Nussenblatt RB, Palestine AG, Chan CC, et al. Effectiveness of cyclosporin therapy for Behcet's disease. Arthritis Rheum 1985;28:671–679
27. Yazici H, Pazarli H, Barnes CG, et al. A controlled trial of azathioprine in Behçet's syndrome. N Engl J Med 1990;322:281–285
28. Rosenbaum JT. Bilateral anterior uveitis and interstitial nephritis. Am J Ophthalmol 1988;105:534–537
29. Garry RF, Fermin CD, Hart DJ, et al. Detection of a human intracisternal A-type retroviral particle antigenically related to HIV. Science 1990;250:1127–1129
30. Rosenbaum JT, Bennett RM. Chronic anterior and posterior uveitis and primary Sjögren's syndrome. Am J Ophthalmol 1987;104:346–352
31. Chan CC, Palestine AG, Kuwabara T, Nussenblatt RB. Immunopathologic study of Vogt-Koyanagi-Harada syndrome. Am J Ophthalmol 1988;105:607–611
32. Landing BH, Larson EJ. Are infantile periarteritis nodosa with coronary artery involvement and fatal mucocutaneous lymph node syndrome the same? Comparison of 20 patients from North America with patients from Hawaii and Japan. Pediatrics 1977;59:651–662
33. Burke MJ, Rennebohm RM. Eye involvement in Kawasaki disease. J Pediatr Ophthalmol Strabismus 1981;18:7–11
34. Porter R. Uveitis in association with multiple sclerosis. Br J Ophthalmol 1988; 56:478–481
35. Meisler DM, Tomsak RL, Khoury S, et al. Anterior uveitis and multiple sclerosis. Cleve Clin J Med 1989;56:535–538
36. Smith RE, Nozik RA. Viruses and atypical bacteria as causes of uveitis. In: Uveitis: a clinical approach to diagnosis and management. Baltimore: Williams & Wilkins, 1983:173–175
37. Shields JA, Waring GO, Monte LG. Ocular findings in leprosy. Am J Ophthalmol 1974;77:880–890
38. Tilden ME, Rosenbaum JT, Fraunfelder FT. Systemic sulfonamides as a cause of bilateral, anterior uveitis. Arch Ophthalmol 1991;109:67–69
39. Rosenthal AR. Ocular manifestations of leukemia. Ophthalmology 1983;90: 899–905
40. Gold DH, Morris DA, Henkind P. Ocular findings in systemic lupus erythematosus. Br J Ophthalmol 1972;56:800–804
41. Haynes BF, Fishman ML, Fauci AS, Wolff SM. The ocular manifestations of Wegener's granulomatosis. Am J Med 1977;63:131–141
42. Passo MS, Rosenbaum JT. Ocular syphilis in patients with human immunodeficiency virus infection. Am J Ophthalmol 1988;106:1–6
43. Aaberg TM. The expanding ophthalmologic spectrum of Lyme disease. Am J Ophthalmol 1989;107:77–80
44. Isaak BL, Liesegang TJ, Michet CJ Jr. Ocular and systemic findings in relapsing polychondritis. Ophthalmology 1986;93:681–689
45. Case records of the Massachusetts General Hospital (Case 2-1990). N Engl J Med 1990;322:116–123

Systemic Associations of Exophthalmos

Hector M. Marines, M.D.
James R. Patrinely, M.D.

Exophthalmos is one of the most common clinical manifestations of orbital disease. The term *exophthalmos* refers to the abnormal anterior displacement of the eye that usually results from a space-occupying abnormality, inflammatory process, or any condition that narrows the orbital cavity. The terms *exophthalmos* and *ocular proptosis* are used interchangeably, although some clinicians use *exophthalmos* exclusively to describe ocular proptosis associated with dysthyroid orbitopathy.

Exophthalmos is usually associated with a variety of signs (globe displacement, eyelid edema, etc.) and symptoms (diplopia, pain, etc.) that will lead the clinician toward a possible diagnosis. The direction of the eye displacement, for example, may reflect the location of the lesion. Thus, space-occupying lesions located at the orbital apex, such as optic nerve tumors, will cause axial proptosis, whereas lacrimal gland lesions in the superotemporal fossa will usually produce inferonasal displacement of the globe. Lesions that are extraorbital (i.e., preseptal) usually do not cause exophthalmos unless there is posterior extension into the orbit.

Some entities may cause a false or apparent prominence of the eye, referred to as *pseudoexophthalmos,* which is not associated with tumor, inflammatory processes, or vascular disorders. Among the main causes of pseudoexophthalmos are high myopia, eyelid retraction, increased scleral show, and contralateral enophthalmos.

The purpose of this chapter is to provide a review of the various systemic diseases that may produce exophthalmos at some point during the course of the disease by involving orbital tissues (Table). Such diseases will be associated with various patterns of orbital involvement (Fig 1), and knowledge of these patterns may allow the clinician to play a key role in the diagnosis and management of these disorders.

Systemic Diseases That May Be Associated with Exophthalmos

Endocrine disorders
Graves' ophthalmopathy
Hypothyroidism
Acromegaly
Cushing's syndrome
Hyperparathyroidism

Lymphoid and hematological disorders
Malignant lymphoma
Multiple myeloma
Leukemia

Histiocytic disorders
Langerhans' cell histiocytosis (histiocytosis X)
 Eosinophilic granuloma
 Letterer-Siwe disease
 Hand-Schüller-Christian disease
Juvenile xanthogranuloma
Sinus histiocytosis with massive lymphadenopathy
Erdheim-Chester disease (systemic xanthogranulomatosis)

Noninfectious orbital inflammation
Sarcoidosis
Multifocal fibrosclerosis
Systemic lupus erythematosus
Dermatomyositis
Giant-cell polymyositis
Wegener's granulomatosis
Polyarteritis nodosa
Cogan's syndrome (atypical form)
Lethal midline granuloma
Angiolymphoid hyperplasia with eosinophilia (Kimura's disease)
Amyloidosis

Infectious orbital inflammation
Pyemic cellulitis
Tuberculosis
Syphilis
Mucormycosis
Aspergillosis
Echinococcosis (hydatid disease)
Trichinosis
Amebiasis
Lyme disease

Fibroosseous lesions
Fibrous dysplasia and Albright's syndrome
Brown tumor in hyperparathyroidism
Orbital osteomas in Gardner's syndrome
Multiple enchondromatosis (Ollier's disease)
Infantile cortical hyperostosis (Caffey's disease)
Hereditary diaphyseal dysplasia (Engelmann's disease)
Osteopetrosis (Albers-Schönberg disease)

Phakomatoses
Neurofibromatosis
Wyburn-Mason syndrome

continued

Systemic Diseases That May Be Associated with Exophthalmos (continued)

Phakomatoses (cont.)
Osler-Weber-Rendu syndrome
Klippel-Trenaunay-Weber syndrome
Sturge-Weber syndrome

Metastatic tumors to the orbit
In children
- Neuroblastoma
- Ewing's sarcoma
- Wilms' tumor
- Medulloblastoma
- Sarcoma
- Other cancers

In adults
- Breast adenocarcinoma
- Lung cancer
- Prostate cancer
- Gastrointestinal tract cancer
- Renal cell cancer
- Thyroid cancer
- Melanoma
- Carcinoid
- Other cancers

Congenital craniofacial deformities
Crouzon's disease
Apert's syndrome
Pfeiffer's syndrome
Kleeblattschädel anomaly
Lowry syndrome
Hermann-Optiz syndrome
Sakati-Nyhan-Tisdale syndrome
Other craniofacial disorders

■ Endocrine Disorders

Graves' Ophthalmopathy

The most common cause of exophthalmos in adults, either unilaterally or bilaterally, is dysthyroid ophthalmopathy. The systemic manifestations of hyperthyroidism include weight loss, fatigue, sweating, irritability, heat intolerance, and palpitations, all due to increased triiodothyronine (T_3) and thyroxine (T_4). Discussion of the metabolic changes in hyperthyroidism are beyond the scope of this chapter.

Graves' disease is by far the most common form of hyperthyroidism and consists of a classical triad of major manifestations: hyperthyroidism with diffuse goiter, ophthalmopathy, and infiltrative dermopathy (pretibial myxedema). These manifestations do not necessarily appear together.

The ophthalmic manifestations of thyroid dysfunction are referred to as *Graves' ophthalmopathy*. Some other terms have been used interchangeably in the literature with Graves' ophthalmopathy, including *dysthyroid ophthalmopathy*,

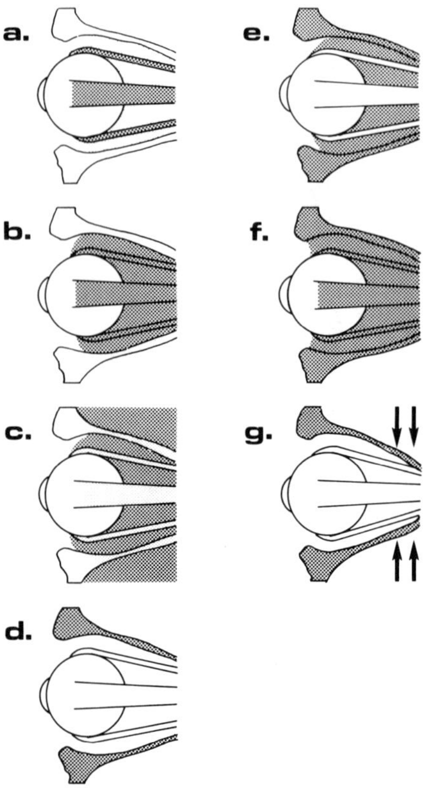

Figure 1 *Patterns of orbital involvement in systemic conditions producing exophthalmos. Primary areas of involvement are dark-shaded and secondary areas of involvement are light-shaded: (a) endocrine disorders (primary—muscles; secondary—soft tissues); (b) lymphoid, hematological, and noninfectious inflammation (all orbital tissues except bone); (c) infectious inflammation (primary—paranasal sinuses and orbital soft tissues; secondary—bone and muscles); (d) fibroosseous lesions (primary—bone); (e) histiocytic disorders (primary—orbital soft tissues and bone); (f) metastatic tumors (all orbital tissues and bone); and (g) congenital craniofacial deformities (showing decreased orbital volume).*

dysthyroid orbitopathy, endocrine exophthalmos, Graves' orbitopathy, infiltrative ophthalmopathy, thyroid eye disease, and *malignant exophthalmos.*

The common manifestations of Graves' ophthalmopathy include upper and lower eyelid retraction, lagophthalmos, conjunctival chemosis, restriction of eye movement manifested as diplopia, eyelid edema, and axial exophthalmos (Fig 2). Most of these findings are related to swelling of the orbital tissues, predominantly the extraocular muscles and orbital fat from lymphoplasmacytic infiltration, mucopolysaccharide deposition, and fatty degeneration. This may lead to muscle enlargement and fibrosis, with subsequent motility disturbances, and possible visual loss due to compression of the optic nerve at the orbital apex, which occurs in 2 to 5% of the cases [1]. The inferior and medial recti muscles are the most commonly affected. The pathogenesis of Graves' ophthalmopathy remains uncertain, although an immunological mechanism is strongly supported from data in the literature [2–4].

Due to the unclear pathogenesis of Graves' ophthalmopathy, universal principles of management have not been established. Primarily, good control of the hyperthyroidism must be achieved, although Graves' ophthalmopathy does not necessarily behave parallel to the thyroid state [5].

Exophthalmos itself is not an indication for either medical or surgical

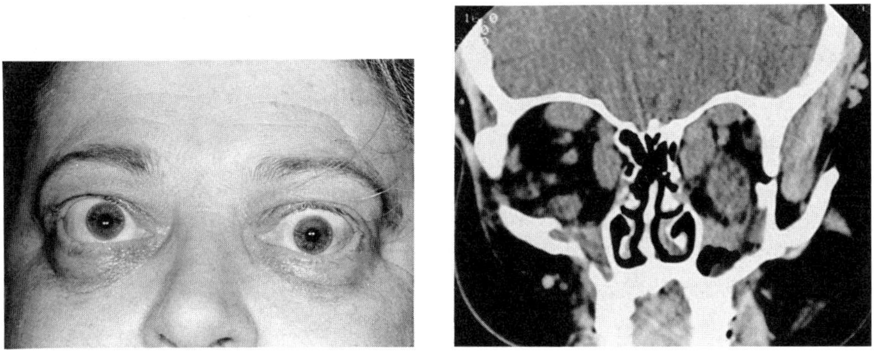

Figure 2 *(A) Patient with severe Graves' (dysthyroid) ophthalmopathy demonstrating bilateral exophthalmos, dysconjugate strabismus, and eyelid retraction. (B) Coronal computed tomography scan of same patient after orbital decompression (ethmoidectomy and maxillary antrostomy), displaying typical marked enlargement of extraocular muscles seen prolapsing into sinus cavities.*

treatment unless it is sight-threatening or cosmetically unacceptable, although supportive care and close observation may be necessary. Exposure due to severe proptosis and compressive optic neuropathy are the major indications for orbital decompression [6].

Surgical management of Graves' ophthalmopathy, when indicated, includes orbital decompression, muscle surgery, upper or lower eyelid retraction correction and, occasionally, blepharoplasty. The role of noninvasive modalities such as systemic corticosteroids and radiotherapy is variable. A good to excellent response (relief of congestion and visual improvement) in 70% of patients treated with irradiation has been reported by Rootman [7], although exophthalmos and motility dysfunctions responded only moderately.

Hypothyroidism

Chronic autoimmune thyroiditis and radioiodine therapy for hyperthyroidism are the most common causes of primary hypothyroidism. Other causes include external radiotherapy, thyroidectomy, thyroid gland dysgenesis, and others. Secondary hypothyroidism is due to pituitary or hypothalamic disease. Cretinism, which is a result of a deficiency of thyroid hormone during fetal or early life, is encountered in children and infants. Causes of this deficiency include dysgenesis of the thyroid gland, metabolic errors, and chronic iodine deficiency in regions where goiter is endemic. Systemic manifestations will vary depending on the form of hypothyroidism (i.e., cretinism, adulthood hypothyroidism).

It is important to distinguish between hypothyroidism associated with Graves' disease and primary hypothyroidism. Exophthalmos is commonly seen in the euthyroid or hypothyroid patient following treatment for hyperthyroidism. In other forms of hypothyroidism, however, exophthalmos is an unusual feature [8]. Although the pathogenetic mechanism is unclear, orbital edema due to deposition of mucopolysaccharides may explain the proptosis rarely seen in primary hypothyroidism.

Acromegaly

Acromegaly is another endocrinological disorder in which exophthalmos is a potential manifestation as a result of enlarged extraocular muscles [9]. We are not aware, however, of any report in the literature of exophthalmos as a feature of acromegaly.

Cushing's Syndrome

Exophthalmos can also be associated with exogenous and endogenous Cushing's syndrome [10, 11]. A steroid-induced increase of the orbital fat seems to be the mechanism for the exophthalmos. This has been supported by computed tomography findings in several series [10, 12]. The pathophysiology of the orbital fat changes has not been well elucidated, although a differential binding of glucocorticoids to adipose tissue receptors and an enhancement of lipoprotein lipase activity has been strongly supported [13].

Hyperparathyroidism

Hyperparathyroidism is another endocrinological disorder that can present with exophthalmos and will be discussed in the section on fibroosseous lesions.

■ Lymphoid and Hematological Disorders

Lymphoid tumors and leukemias represent an important group among the systemic diseases that involve the orbit, with proptosis as a major clinical manifestation.

Lymphoma

The great majority of lymphoid lesions involving the orbit are of the non-Hodgkin's variety. Histopathologically, these lesions may be classified as benign reactive lymphoid hyperplasia, atypical lymphoid hyperplasia, and malignant lymphoma. For purposes of this discussion, malignant lymphoma is highlighted since it is the only one that usually occurs as a systemic disorder. Although lymphoma may occur primarily in the orbit, the incidence of orbital involvement in systemic lymphoma is considered to be rather low (1.3%) [14], with the predominance of cases occurring in adulthood. Lymphomalike lesions of the orbit in children should be considered as a manifestation of leukemia, except for Burkitt's lymphoma, which is a rapidly growing tumor seen more commonly in African children. Some cases of Burkitt's lymphoma have been reported in Americans [15] and associated with the acquired immunodeficiency syndrome (AIDS) [16].

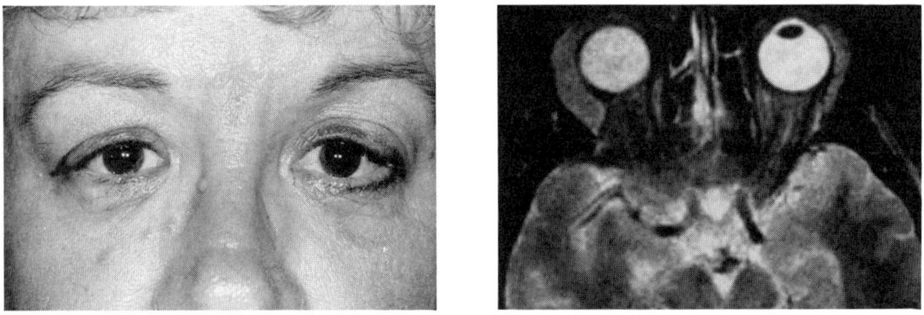

A B

Figure 3 *(A) Patient with systemic lymphoma demonstrating bilateral, diffuse, firm swelling of upper eyelids and left proptosis. There were also fleshy subconjunctival deposits present (not shown in photograph). (B) Axial magnetic resonance imaging scan of same patient showing bilateral orbital involvement in area of lacrimal gland. The well-defined orbital mass conforms to globe and orbital bones, representing lymphomatous infiltration.*

The presentation of orbital malignant lymphoma is often proptosis with downward displacement of the eye due to the tendency of this neoplasm to involve the superior orbit (Fig 3). Anterior involvement is also common, manifested by subconjunctival lesions described as "salmon patches" due to their peculiar pinkish coloration. In cases of Burkitt's lymphoma, exophthalmos is more pronounced and develops more rapidly.

Another type of systemic lymphoma is large-cell lymphoma, also called *histiocytic lymphoma.* This form has a characteristic clinical presentation with eyelid edema and puffiness followed by proptosis. In 50% of cases, the orbital involvement is the initial presentation. A similar clinical picture may also be observed in orbital involvement of cutaneous T-cell lymphoma (mycosis fungoides) [17, 18].

Hodgkin's disease is very rare in the orbit [19, 20]. When it does occur, it is usually in advanced systemic disease, presenting with clinical manifestations similar to those of any lymphoid disorder.

Multiple Myeloma

Another group of neoplasms capable of involving the orbit are the lymphoplasmacytic tumors. Of this group, multiple myeloma is most important since it can spread to the orbit as well as to other ocular structures. Orbital involvement in myeloma, although very rare, may be the initial manifestation of the disease [21]. Proptosis with displacement of the eye and subsequent diplopia may be the earliest clinical signs of multiple myeloma. These patients are usually treated with combined chemotherapy and orbital radiation.

Some lymphoplasmacytoid lesions (plasmacytomas) may occur as localized processes in the orbit, unrelated to multiple myeloma.

Waldenström's macroglobulinemia is a lymphoplasmacytoid disorder that resembles multiple myeloma (monoclonal immunoglobulin production) and lymphocytic lymphoma (infiltration of lymphoid tissues) and may involve the orbit as part of a systemic disease, inducing exophthalmos [22].

Leukemia

An important group of disorders that may involve the eye and the orbit consists of the leukemias, which mainly affect children. Although clinical evidence of orbital infiltration with proptosis is rare, it has been assumed that microscopic involvement may be more common. When exophthalmos does occur, it usually evolves rapidly and may present with hemorrhage and ecchymosis due to the alterations in blood supply, vessel fragility, and coagulopathy. Orbital and ocular involvement are more commonly seen in association with acute leukemias and may be bilateral.

Granulocytic sarcoma is a term that refers to orbital infiltration by acute myelocytic leukemia and is the most common form of leukemic infiltration to the orbit [23]. Granulocytic sarcoma often presents prior to hematological evidence of the disease and is bilateral in approximately 10% of the cases, frequently involving the lateral wall of the orbit [24]. Proptosis is often rapidly progressive. Differential diagnosis includes other rapidly growing tumors, such as rhabdomyosarcoma, metastatic neuroblastoma, and Ewing's sarcoma.

Management is usually nonsurgical, with radiotherapy and chemotherapy being the two predominate forms of treatment.

■ Histiocytic Disorders

There is a group of proliferative histiocytic disorders that may involve the orbit either as a localized form or as part of a systemic process. This group includes histiocytosis X (Langerhans' cell histiocytosis), juvenile xanthogranuloma, sinus histiocytosis with massive lymphadenopathy, and Erdheim-Chester disease. Sarcoidosis, although considered a histiocytic disorder, will be discussed in the section on noninfectious orbital inflammation.

Langerhans' Cell Histiocytosis

Langerhans' cell histiocytosis (histiocytosis X), or eosinophilic granuloma, can occur in a localized form or as a disseminated disorder [25]. Eosinophilic granuloma is a disease of children and teenagers and is rarely seen in adults. The multisystem form of eosinophilic granuloma, also known as Letterer-Siwe disease, very seldom involves the eye or the orbit and affects very young children. Hand-Schüller-Christian disease is a variant seen in older children, usually over age 3, and commonly involves the orbit. It presents with a triad of bilateral proptosis, lytic lesions in the cranial bones, and diabetes insipidus. Orbital involvement, however, is more commonly seen in the localized or focal form of eosinophilic granuloma, which more frequently affects the superior or superotemporal orbital bones. Exophthalmos may or may not occur, depending on the degree of orbital involvement, but pain and skin erythema are typically present. Management includes surgical debridement and curettage of orbital lesions, with chemotherapy and radiotherapy recommended for more severe forms [26].

Other Histiocytic Disorders

Juvenile Xanthogranuloma Another histiocytic lesion that may involve the orbit, producing unilateral or bilateral exophthalmos, is juvenile xanthogranuloma. This condition is characterized by granulomatous inflammation more commonly involving the anterior uvea. A few cases have been reported, however, in which orbital involvement occurred [27, 28]. Management includes the use of systemic or locally injected steroids, although no well-defined therapy has been established.

Sinus Histiocytosis with Massive Lymphadenopathy Bilateral or unilateral proptosis, often associated with eyelid edema, can be a manifestation of massive idiopathic infiltration by lymphocytes and histiocytes in the orbital tissues and the cervical and retroperitoneal lymph nodes. This condition is termed *sinus histiocytosis with massive lymphadenopathy*. Several cases have been reported with orbital involvement, usually in the lacrimal gland region, producing inflammatory signs and symptoms [29]. Sinus histiocytosis is usually a self-limited condition.

Erdheim-Chester Disease Erdheim-Chester disease is the systemic form of xanthogranulomatosis (lipoid granulomatosis) that typically affects other organs including kidney, lungs, heart, retroperitoneal tissues, and the orbital soft tissues [30]. Collections of lipid-laden histiocytes intermixed with inflammatory cells are observed in the involved tissues. Bilateral proptosis, associated with xanthelasma lesions of eyelids, is the clinical presentation of Erdheim-Chester disease of the orbit, which may respond to systemic corticosteroids.

■ Noninfectious Orbital Inflammation

Exophthalmos may be seen as a clinical sign of idiopathic inflammatory processes of the orbit, which can be part of a systemic disorder or a more localized disease. Dysthyroid orbitopathy (Graves' ophthalmopathy) is the most important disorder in this group and has been previously reviewed in the section on endocrine disorders (see page 145). Another important entity in this group of idiopathic inflammations is inflammatory pseudotumor of the orbit, although this is a localized entity and not a manifestation of systemic disease. Several noninfectious inflammatory systemic disorders that can cause exophthalmos when involving the orbit have been outlined in the Table, with sarcoidosis being the most important.

Sarcoidosis Sarcoidosis is a multisystem granulomatous disorder of unknown etiology and pathogenesis that can involve almost every organ in the body. Practically every tissue in the eye may also be affected, with a predilection for the uveal tract [31]. Sarcoidosis has a marked tendency to involve the lacrimal gland but very rarely affects the other orbital tissues [32]. Lesions encountered in the orbit that display histological features similar to those of sarcoidosis (noncaseating epithelioid cell granulomas) without systemic manifestations are referred to as *sarcoid,* which may be completely unrelated to systemic sarcoidosis.

Clinical manifestations of ocular sarcoidosis include signs of chronic intraocular and extraocular inflammation as well as enlargement of the lacrimal gland. Lacrimal gland enlargement does not necessarily cause proptosis unless there is more extensive posterior involvement of the orbit. Optic nerve involvement may rarely occur and mimic a primary tumor of the nerve [31]. Specific clinical, laboratory, and radiological signs of systemic sarcoidosis are usually present. The management of ocular and orbital sarcoidosis includes the use of topical and systemic corticosteroids and, occasionally, immunosuppressives.

Multifocal Fibrosclerosis Exophthalmos has also been documented as a manifestation of multifocal fibrosclerosis, a rare idiopathic sclerosing process that may involve the retroperitoneal tissues, mediastinal structures, thyroid gland and, occasionally, the orbit, causing unilateral or bilateral proptosis [33]. A dense diffuse hyalinization of the affected tissues is observed histopathologically.

Connective Tissue Diseases There are few reported cases of systemic lupus erythematosus presenting with exophthalmos [34–36]. Rapidly developing proptosis associated with orbital inflammation and myositis were the clinical and computed tomographic findings in these cases.

Another connective tissue disease associated with exophthalmos is dermatomyositis [37], which can present with iritis, extraocular muscle paralysis, neuritis, and skin inflammation. A nongranulomatous myositis and vasculitis are observed histopathologically.

Painful proptosis with ophthalmoplegia may be present in giant-cell polymyositis. This is a sometimes fatal disease that is manifested by mononuclear and giant-cell inflammation of the myocardium and skeletal muscle [38].

Vasculitides There is a subgroup of vasculitides within the inflammatory group, characterized by destruction of vessels from an immune complex–mediated injury. Of this group, Wegener's granulomatosis is more commonly associated with orbital disease (18–22%). Painful proptosis, signs of inflammation, and congestion are the most common orbital presentations. Differential diagnosis should include idiopathic inflammation of the orbit and malignancy. The systemic manifestations of the disease, including respiratory symptoms and manifestations of multisystemic vasculitis (arthralgias, dermatitis, endocarditis, glomerulonephritis) are usually helpful in making the diagnosis. A tissue biopsy, however, is necessary for diagnostic confirmation. Scleritis, episcleritis, and peripheral corneal ulceration are among the most common ocular manifestations of Wegener's granulomatosis.

Exophthalmos due to necrosis and inflammation of orbital soft tissues secondary to vasculitis with thrombotic occlusion is observed in polyarteritis nodosa. Idiopathic thrombophlebitis may also produce severe signs and symptoms of orbital disease resembling orbital neoplasia [39].

Cogan's syndrome has been reported to present with mild proptosis. This syndrome classically consists of interstitial keratitis, vertigo, and auditory symptoms. There is, however, an atypical form that may present with ocular and orbital involvement. It may be associated with systemic necrotizing vasculitis and present as an orbital cellulitis [40].

Lethal Midline Granuloma Another condition to be considered in this section is idiopathic midline destructive disease, or lethal midline granuloma. The pathogenesis is unknown, although it has been described as a form of lymphoma and may have features of Wegener's granulomatosis. Due to its peculiar location in the midline of the face, it can secondarily extend into the orbit with the resultant signs of orbital disease.

Kimura's Disease The orbit may also be affected as part of a rare disseminated inflammatory disorder that typically involves the skin of the head and neck and is associated with blood and tissue eosinophilia. This entity is termed *angiolymphoid hyperplasia with eosinophilia* or *Kimura's disease.* It frequently affects the superior orbit, causing proptosis with downward displacement of the eyeball. Histopathologically, there is a proliferation of blood vessels and diffuse infiltration of lymphocytes and eosinophils. Complete excision of the lesion is the treatment of choice.

Amyloidosis The last condition to be considered among noninfectious inflammatory diseases is amyloidosis. Although considered by some to be a deposition disorder, it is actually a complex group of conditions of unclear etiology and pathogenesis, characterized by the deposition of fibrillary proteins called *amyloid.* Several forms have been described, including primary and secondary amyloidosis. Furthermore, it may present as a localized or widespread systemic disease. Amyloidosis has been associated with multiple myeloma, lymphoma, chronic inflammation, and other disorders [41–43].

Orbital amyloidosis was observed in 6 patients (16%) of 37 cases reported by Lemke and co-workers [44] and may be observed as a localized process or as a manifestation of systemic amyloidosis. Exophthalmos, however, is not always a presenting sign of orbital amyloidosis and obviously will depend on the degree of amyloid deposition. Eyelid thickening and blepharoptosis are the most common manifestations of amyloidosis of the orbit and adnexa [45]. A tendency for bleeding due to vascular fragility secondary to perivascular involvement is a remarkable characteristic of amyloid infiltration, so spontaneous subconjunctival hemorrhage or eyelid ecchymosis may be the initial presentation.

Surgical debulking of the amyloid deposits may be indicated in symptomatic cases. The prognosis, however, is variable, with improvement or stabilization in some cases and recurrence in others.

■ Infectious Orbital Inflammation

The orbit is very commonly affected by diverse inflammatory systemic processes, as was just reviewed. Inflammatory orbital diseases are by far the most common causes (excluding trauma) of exophthalmos, and infectious orbital inflammatory diseases are a major component.

Orbital infection, which very rarely arises spontaneously in the orbit, is generally secondary to infection spreading from adjacent structures including the sinuses, brain, and eyelids. Orbital infection arising from hematogenous seeding as a manifestation of systemic disease is, however, very rare [46]. The most common form of orbital infectious inflammation is that associated with infectious sinus disease [46]. This can be caused by bacteria and fungi, particularly those of the class Phycomycetes *(Mucor)* and species from the genus *Aspergillus*. Orbital inflammation related to sinus disease is considered a local process and not a systemic disorder and is, therefore, beyond the context of this discussion. It should be mentioned, however, that mucormycosis of the orbit is frequently observed in poorly controlled diabetes with ketoacidosis, presenting with proptosis, painful ophthalmoplegia, and marked necrosis of the orbital tissues (Fig 4). Management of mucormycosis includes wide surgical debridement of devitalized tissue as well as systemic and local amphotericin. Benefit may be derived from hyperbaric oxygen therapy [47].

Pyemic Cellulitis

Pyemic cellulitis is a form of orbital cellulitis that can result from bacteremia in a compromised host. This form of cellulitis is often caused by unusual organisms, and its clinical presentation is similar to that of orbital inflammation associated with sinus infection.

Other Infections

Infectious granulomatous inflammation of the orbit rarely occurs but may be due to tuberculosis [48], syphilis [49], and some fungi. Occasionally, parasites (see the Table) can also invade the soft tissues of the orbit with a variety of clinical manifestations [50–52].

Lyme disease has been reported to cause orbital myositis with exophthalmos [53]. Clinical signs such as erythema chronicum migrans and other organ involvement are important to diagnose Lyme disease, which is caused by the spirochete *Borrelia burgdorferi* found in deer ticks. Treatment is with systemic antibiotics.

A patient with amebiasis of the gastrointestinal tract who developed proptosis was reported by Jakobiec and Jones [49]. Although no organisms were obtained from the orbital tissues, resolution of the proptosis was observed with antiamebic treatment.

■ Fibroosseous Lesions

Some systemic disorders may present with orbital lesions that originate in osseous, chondroid, or fibroosseous structures. From this group, *fibrous dysplasia* is the most common one affecting the orbital bones and is caused by an idiopathic arrest in bone maturation. This disorder usually develops in children during the first or second decades of life. It may present as an isolated orbital form (monostotic) or as a systemic multifocal (polyostotic) disease sometimes involving the orbit (Fig 5). When the polyostotic form is associated with café-au-lait spots and endocrine dysfunction (precocious puberty), it is known as *Albright's syndrome*. This syndrome occurs in girls and rarely involves the orbit [54]. The clinical orbital manifestations will vary, depending on the bones affected. The usual presentation is facial deformity, mild exophthalmos, and

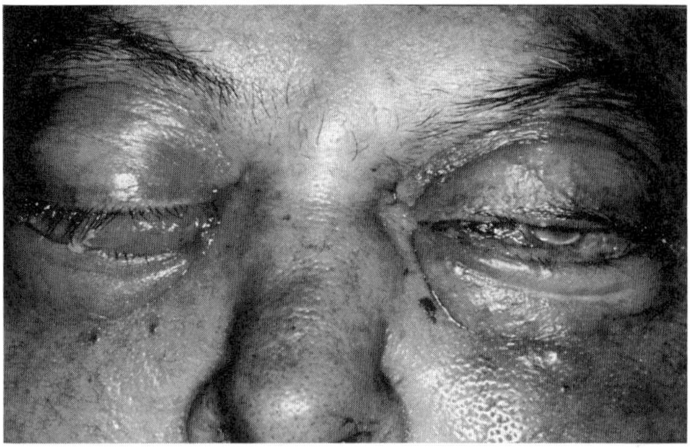

A

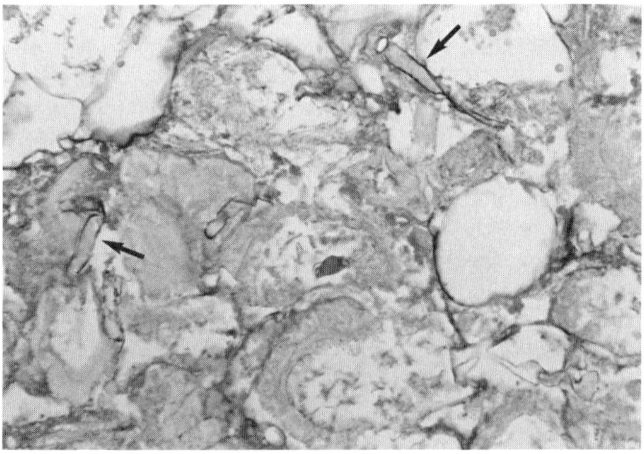

B

Figure 4 *(A) Signs of periorbital inflammation with bilateral proptosis. Ophthalmoplegia and loss of vision in a patient with uncontrolled diabetes mellitus who developed mucormycosis of the orbits and sinuses. (B) Left orbital exenteration specimen displayed broad, branching, nonseptate organisms (hematoxylin-eosin) consistent with the diagnosis of mucormycosis.*

inferior displacement of the eyeball due to the frequent involvement of the frontal bone. Decreased vision should suggest the possibility of optic nerve compression via canal stenosis, which is the most serious ocular complication of fibrous dysplasia. Surgical debulking may be indicated if the lesion is cosmetically unacceptable or signs of optic nerve compression appear. The use of radiotherapy is controversial due to the possible induction of malignant changes (osteogenic sarcoma).

Another lesion in this category, although rare, is the *brown tumor* of the orbit associated with *hyperparathyroidism* [55]. This tumor usually presents as a palpable mass with painful exophthalmos and motility disturbances and is be-

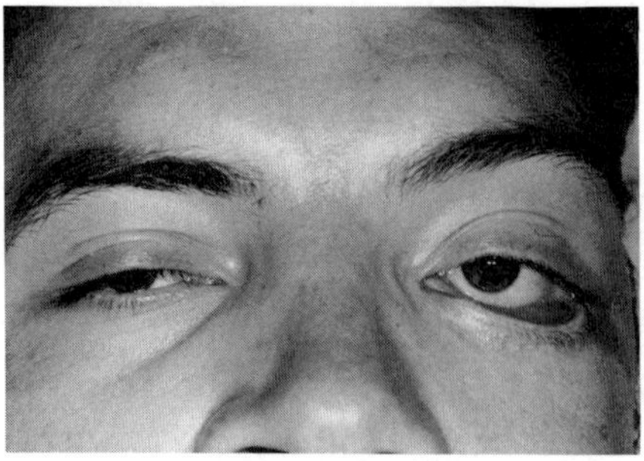

Figure 5 *Patient with fibrous dysplasia involving the left orbital bones (polyostotic) showing facial asymmetry with proptosis and medial displacement of eye. Left lower eyelid retraction is also present.*

lieved to be a form of reactive replacement of bone by fibrous tissue [56]. Surgical excision is the treatment of choice, combined with control of hyperparathyroidism.

Multiple osteomas can be observed among the manifestations of *Gardner's syndrome,* a condition characterized by familial intestinal polyposis and a higher incidence of carcinoma of the colon. Osteomas in Gardner's syndrome may at times involve the orbital bones, inducing proptosis [57]. Exophthalmos has been reported as an early clinical manifestation in this syndrome [58]. Surgical management of the osteomas is advised in large symptomatic tumors. Small lesions may be followed closely.

DeLaey and colleagues [59] reported orbital involvement in multiple enchondromatosis, also called *Ollier's disease.* This is a rare idiopathic disorder characterized by chondroid tumors. The long bones are particularly involved, with occasional occurrence in the ethmoid sinus and extension into the orbit. The clinical picture is that of sinusitis with exophthalmos. Radiotherapy is usually effective in the treatment of this disorder. Systemic enchondromatosis may be associated with soft-tissue hemangiomas (Maffucci's syndrome), which may involve the orbit [60].

A disease rarely seen by ophthalmologists is *infantile cortical hyperostosis* (Caffey's disease) characterized by swelling of the soft tissues of the face, jaws, and periocular region, usually causing proptosis [61]. The onset of the disorder is in the first weeks of life and basically consists of inflammation affecting the periosteum and secondary hyperplasia of the cortical bone. In the differential diagnosis, the primary distinction to be made is between Caffey's disease and osteogenic sarcoma. Most of the cases resolve with nonspecific supportive treatment.

Progressive hereditary diaphyseal dysplasia, also known as *Engelmann's disease,* is a rare idiopathic bone dystrophy associated with osteosclerosis. Among the most common clinical manifestations are pain in the extremities, fatigability, neuromuscular weakness with poor musculature, hypogonadism with delayed puberty, and dry skin. The orbital involvement includes papilledema with optic atrophy and exophthalmos [62]. Biopsy of the affected bones shows periosteal thickening with cortical and endosteal hyperostosis. There is no specific therapy for this disorder, and surgical orbital decompression may be indicated when there is evidence of compressive optic neuropathy.

Also considered among this group of fibroosseous lesions is *Albers-*

Schönberg disease or *osteopetrosis*. This is a rare congenital disease characterized by extensive osteosclerosis as a result of a defect in bone metabolism with osteoclastic cell dysfunction (inadequate bone resorption). Benign (autosomal dominant) and malignant (autosomal recessive) forms have been described, according to the clinical course of the disease. The most common ocular manifestation of osteopetrosis is optic atrophy resulting from narrowing of the optic foramen. Early surgical decompression is indicated in these cases. Exophthalmos and exotropia secondary to shallow orbits have been reported in 25% of the cases of osteopetrosis [63]. Retinal degeneration and nasolacrimal duct obstruction are also seen. Other manifestations of this bone disorder include cranial neuropathy, pathological fractures, dwarfism, frontal bossing, and large head. Management is mainly symptomatic in the benign forms. Calcitrol and bone marrow transplantation have been reported successful in the management of the recessive form [64].

■ Phakomatoses

There is a group of systemic diseases, termed *phakomatoses,* characterized by the presence of hamartomatous lesions that involve different tissues and often ocular structures. Neurofibromatosis, also termed *von Recklinghausen's disease,* is probably the most common disease involving the orbit and occurs in a variety of forms. Neurofibromatosis Type I (NF-1) is the principal form, whereas neurofibromatosis Type II (NF-2) is associated with bilateral acoustic neuromas. The classical lesion is the plexiform neurofibroma that originates from peripheral nerves in the orbit, causing bony changes and thickening of periocular tissues. Facial disfigurement and exophthalmos with inferior globe displacement may occur. The proptosis may be pulsatile when there is marked hypoplasia of the orbital walls, particularly the greater wing of the sphenoid. Because of the diffuse infiltrating nature of this tumor, complete surgical excision is practically impossible. Surgical debulking should be limited to cases where symptoms or cosmetic problems make it necessary. Other causes of exophthalmos in neurofibromatosis include the development of optic nerve gliomas, meningiomas, and schwannomas.

Wyburn-Mason syndrome is the other phakomatosis of interest since it may include orbital arteriovenous malformations that may present clinically as pulsating proptosis with decreased vision. Similar findings have been reported in rare cases of Osler-Weber-Rendu syndrome and in the Klippel-Trenaunay-Weber syndrome, in which orbital varices have been discovered [65].

Orbital involvement in encephalotrigeminal angiomatosis (Sturge-Weber syndrome) is unusual. However, there are reports of vascular malformations causing exophthalmos in this syndrome [66].

■ Metastatic Tumors

Metastatic tumors of the orbit account for 2 to 10% of orbital tumors. Metastases reach the orbit only by hematogenous routes since lymphatics are normally not present in the orbital tissues. Orbital metastases occur less frequently than uveal metastases [67, 68]. In a study of 210 patients with uveal metastases, 35 were found to have orbital metastatic disease as well [68].

When discussing metastatic tumors to the orbit, a distinction between children and adults should be made since different tumors predominate in these age groups. Neuroblastoma arising from the adrenal medulla is the most common metastatic tumor in children, followed by Ewing's sarcoma, Wilms' tumor, medulloblastoma, and sarcomas. In adults, carcinomas are the most common metastatic neoplasms, with breast adenocarcinoma being the most frequent, followed by lung, prostate, and gastrointestinal tract cancer.

Rapidly progressive proptosis and displacement of the eye combined with secondary functional alterations reflecting the location and characteristics of the tumor account for the main clinical manifestations of metastatic tumors. Diplopia, due to muscle abnormalities either neurological or restrictive, as well as some other signs such as blepharoptosis or manifestations of sensory dysfunction (e.g., decrease of vision, pain, or paresthesia) are also commonly observed. Bilateral involvement is present in 14% of the cases [69].

Although exophthalmos is one of the major signs of metastatic neoplasms, enophthalmos can occur as an unusual manifestation and is due to cicatrization and retraction of extraocular muscles and orbital tissues. Enophthalmos is usually associated with scirrhous breast carcinoma, although this sign is not exclusive to this tumor; some other tumors, such as neuroblastoma, may undergo necrosis and hemorrhagic changes presenting with the acute onset of proptosis, eyelid ecchymosis, and inflammation, followed by enophthalmos.

Management of metastatic orbital tumors includes diagnostic surgical biopsy of the lesion followed, in most cases, by radiotherapy and chemotherapy. When dealing with tumors of more aggressive behavior and a tendency to early spreading, wide surgical excision may be recommended.

■ Craniofacial Disorders

Congenital craniofacial abnormalities may initially present to the ophthalmologist. Numerous congenital abnormalities involving the face and cranium have been described, and multiple classifications have been offered. We will review the craniofacial disorders that most frequently disturb the orbital anatomy, with exophthalmos as a common sign. The craniofacial anomalies that involve the orbit may be separated in two groups: (1) the craniosynostoses, or premature closure of cranial sutures, and (2) the clefting syndromes. From these two categories, the craniosynostoses are the ones usually associated with exophthalmos, which is related to variable degrees of volume decrease of the orbital cavity (see Fig 2). Crouzon's disease, Apert's syndrome, and Pfeiffer's syndromes are probably the most common disorders. A variety of cranial deformities can result from premature synostosis including plagiocephaly, brachycephaly, scaphocephaly, oxicephaly, and trigonocephaly. Facial findings associated with craniosynostosis can be observed in various degrees including orbital dystopia, exophthalmos, strabismus, maxillary and zygomatic hypoplasia, and malocclusion. Crouzon's disease is an autosomal dominant disorder characterized by premature craniosynostosis with various cranial vault deformities (brachycephaly is most common), midfacial hypoplasia, and shallow or-

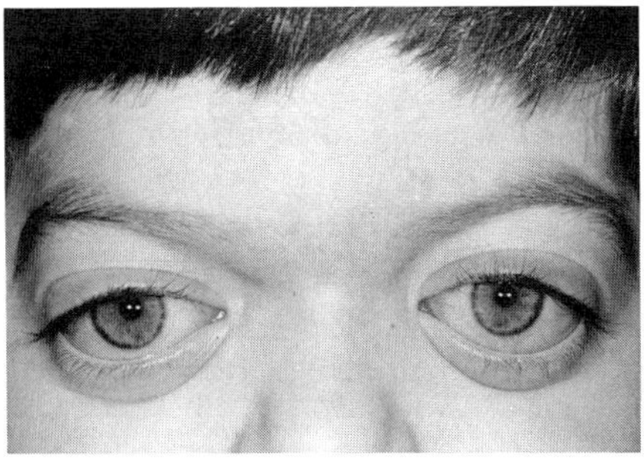

Figure 6 *Crouzon's disease displaying typical midfacial hypoplasia with shallow orbits resulting in marked exophthalmos, hypertelorism, and midface retrusion.*

bits with orbital hypertelorism and exophthalmos as a constant and remarkable feature (Fig 6) [70]. Other classical manifestations of Crouzon's disease are "parrot-beak" nose, cleft palate, and prognathous mandible with severe dental occlusion defects. A wide variety of ocular manifestations may occur in this syndrome. Optic nerve complications (optic atrophy or papilledema) are seen in 25 to 80% of cases [70]. Muscular imbalance, mainly V-pattern exodeviation, is commonly seen with an incidence of approximately 60% [71]. Some other less frequent ocular anomalies have been reported in association with Crouzon's disease, such as aniridia, cataracts, and glaucoma.

Similar findings to those described for Crouzon's disease, associated with syndactyly of the hands and feet, are encountered in Apert's syndrome. This is an autosomal dominant disorder that occurs in approximately 1:160,000 births. Sporadic cases (new mutations) have been found related to advanced paternal age [72]. The craniofacial clinical findings are usually less pronounced than in Crouzon's disease. Other systemic but less frequent abnormalities have been reported to be associated with this syndrome [73].

Other craniosynostoses may also present with orbital abnormalities and exophthalmos but are less frequently seen than Crouzon's disease and Apert's syndrome (see the Table). From this group we will mention only Pfeiffer's syndrome, which is similar to Crouzon's and Apert's with some additional characteristic features including long, broad thumbs and great toes, and varus deformity.

Management of these syndromes requires complicated craniofacial reconstruction and rehabilitation and should be approached by an experienced multidisciplinary craniofacial surgical team.

This research was supported in part by an unrestricted grant to Baylor College of Medicine from Research to Prevent Blindness, Inc., New York, NY.

■ References

1. Trobe JD, Glaser JS, Laflamme P. Dysthyroid optic neuropathy. Arch Ophthalmol 1978;96:1199–1209

2. Char DH. Thyroid eye disease, ed 2. New York: Churchill Livingstone, 1989:95–99
3. Kriss JP, Koniski J, Herman MM. Studies on the pathogenesis of Graves' ophthalmopathy. Recent Prog Horm Res 1975;31:533–566
4. Volpe R. Immunoregulation in autoimmune thyroid disease. N Engl J Med 1987;316:44–45
5. Hamilton HE, Schultz RO, DeGowin EL. Endocrine eye lesion in hyperthyroidism. Arch Intern Med 1960;105:675–685
6. Linberg JV, Anderson RL. Transorbital decompression: indications and results. Arch Ophthalmol 1981;99:113–119
7. Rootman J. Diseases of the orbit. Philadelphia: Lippincott, 1988:262–277
8. Fox R. Infiltrative ophthalmopathy in primary hypothyroidism. Ann Intern Med 1967;67:377–380
9. Patrinely JR, Osborn AG, Anderson RL, Whiting AS. Computed tomographic features of nonthyroid extraocular muscle enlargement. Ophthalmology 1989;96:1038–1047
10. Katz B, Carmody R. Exophthalmos induced by exogenous steroids. J Clin Neuro Ophthalmol 1986;6(4):250–253
11. Haas JS, Nootens RH. Glaucoma secondary to benign adrenal adenoma. Am J Ophthalmol 1974;78:497–500
12. Peyster RG, Ginsberg F, Silber JH, Alder LP. Exophthalmos caused by excessive fat: CT volumetric analysis and differential diagnosis. AJNR 1986;7:35–40
13. De Gasquet P, Pequignot-Planche E, Tonnu NT, Diaby F. Effect of glucocorticoids on lipoprotein lipase activity in rat heart and adipose tissue. Horm Metab Res 1975;7:152–157
14. Rosenberg SA, Diamond HD, Jaslowitz B, Craver LF. Lymphosarcoma: a review of 1269 cases. Medicine (Baltimore) 1961;40:31–84
15. Judson SC, Henle W, Henle G. A cluster of Epstein-Barr virus–associated American Burkitt's lymphoma. N Engl J Med 1977;297:464–468
16. Brooks HL, Downing J, McClure JA, Engel HM. Orbital Burkitt's lymphoma in a homosexual man with acquired immune deficiency. Arch Ophthalmol 1984;102:1533–1537
17. Meekins B, Proia AL, Klintworth GK. Cutaneous T-cell lymphoma presenting as a rapidly enlarging ocular adnexal tumor. Ophthalmology 1985;92:1288–1293
18. Whitbeck EG, Spiers ASD, Hussain M. Mycosis fungoides: subcutaneous and visceral tumors, orbital involvement, and ophthalmoplegia. J Clin Oncol 1983;1:270–276
19. Fratkin JD, Shammas HF, Miller SD. Disseminated Hodgkin's disease with bilateral orbital involvement. Arch Ophthalmol 1978;96:102–104
20. Patel S, Rootman J. Nodular sclerosing Hodgkin's disease of the orbit. Ophthalmology 1983;90:1433–1436
21. Rodman HI, Font RL. Orbital involvement in multiple myeloma. Review of the literature and report of three cases. Arch Ophthalmol 1972;87:30–35
22. Jakobiec FA, McClean I, Font R. Clinicopathologic characteristics of orbital lymphoid hyperplasia. Ophthalmology 1979;86:948–966
23. Zimmerman LE, Font RL. Ophthalmologic manifestations of granulocytic sarcoma (myeloid sarcoma or chloroma). Am J Ophthalmol 1975;80:975–990
24. Shields JA. Diagnosis and management of orbital tumors. Philadelphia: Saunders, 1986:334–336
25. Lichtenstein L. Histiocytosis X. Integration of eosinophilic granuloma of bone "Letterer-Siwe disease" and "Schuller-Christian disease" as related manifestations of a single nosological entity. Arch Pathol 1953;56:84–102
26. Lieberman PH. Eosinophilic granuloma and related syndromes. In: Beeson PB,

McDermott W, Wyngaarden JB, eds. Cecil textbook of medicine, ed 15. Philadelphia: Saunders, 1979:1850–1851

27. Gaynes PM, Cohen GS. Juvenile xanthogranuloma of the orbit. Am J Ophthalmol 1967;63:755–757
28. Sanders TE, Miller JE. Infantile xanthogranuloma of the orbit: report of a case. Trans Am Acad Ophthalmol Otolaryngol 1965;69:458–464
29. Friendly DS, Font RL, Rao NA. Orbital involvement in "sinus" histiocytosis. A report of four cases. Arch Ophthalmol 1977;95:2006–2011
30. Alper MG, Zimmerman LE, LaPiana FG. Orbital manifestations of Erdheim-Chester disease. Trans Am Ophthalmol Soc 1983;81:64–85
31. Obernauf CD, Shaw HE, Sydnor CF, Klintworth GK. Sarcoidosis and its ophthalmic manifestations. Am J Ophthalmol 1978;86:648–655
32. Collison JMT, Miller NR, Green WR. Involvement of orbital tissues by sarcoid. Am J Ophthalmol 1986;102:297–301
33. Richards AB, Skalka HW, Roberts FJ, Flint A. Pseudotumor of the orbit and retroperitoneal fibrosis. A form of multifocal fibrosclerosis. Arch Ophthalmol 1980; 98:1617–1620
34. Grimson BS, Simons KB. Orbital inflammation, myositis and systemic lupus erythematosus. Arch Ophthalmol 1983;101:736–738
35. Brenner EH, Shock JP. Proptosis secondary to systemic lupus erythematosus. Arch Ophthalmol 1974;91:81–82
36. Wilkinson LS, Panusk RS. Exophthalmos associated with systemic lupus erythematosus. Arthritis Rheum 1975;18:188–189
37. Apple DJ, Piest KL. Pathology of selected orbital lesions. In: Smith BC, ed. Ophthalmic plastic and reconstructive surgery. St Louis: Mosby, 1987:1004–1005
38. Kaltah JC, Zimmerman LE, Kolsky MP, Chrousos G, et al. Bilateral orbital involvement in fatal giant cell polymyositis. Ophthalmology 1990;97:520–525
39. Zimmerman LE, Rogers JB. Idiopathic thrombophlebitis of the orbital veins simulating primary tumor of the orbit. Trans Am Acad Ophthalmol Otolaryngol 1957;6:609–613
40. Rootman J. Diseases of the orbit. Philadelphia: Lippincott, 1988:185–193
41. Glenner GG. Amyloid deposits and amyloidosis (pt 1). N Engl J Med 1980;302: 1283–1292
42. Glenner GG. Amyloid deposits and amyloidosis (pt 2). N Engl J Med 1980;302: 1333–1343
43. Glenner GG, Terry WD, Isersky C. Amyloidosis: its nature and pathogenesis. Semin Hematol 1973;10:65–86
44. Lemke BN, Woog JJ, Stasior OG. Amyloidosis of the orbit and adnexa. In: Hornblass A, ed. Oculoplastic orbital and reconstructive surgery, vol 2. Baltimore: Williams & Wilkins, 1990:907–914
45. Smith ME, Zimmerman LE. Amyloidosis of the eyelid and conjunctiva. Arch Ophthalmol 1966;75:42–51
46. Jones DB, Steinkuller PG. Microbial preseptal and orbital cellulitis. In: Tasman W, Jaeger EA, eds. Duane's clinical ophthalmology, vol 4. Philadelphia: Lippincott, 1989:1–24
47. Ferguson BJ, Mitchell TG, Moon R, et al. Adjunctive hyperbaric oxygen for treatment of rhinocerebral mucormycosis. Rev Infect Dis 1988;10:551–559
48. Khaul MK, Lindley S, Matouk E. Tuberculosis of the orbit. Ophthalmology 1985; 92:1624–1627
49. Jakobiec FA, Jones IS. Orbital inflammations. In: Tasman W, Jaeger EA, eds. Duane's clinical ophthalmology, vol 2. Philadelphia: Lippincott, 1989:60–63
50. Binford CH, Connor DH. Pathology of tropical and extraordinary diseases: atlas, vols 1 and 2. Washington: Armed Forces Institute of Pathology, 1976

51. Morales AG, Croxatto JO, Crovetto L, Ebner R. Hydatid cysts of the orbit. A review of 35 cases. Ophthalmology 1988;95:1027–1032
52. Jakobiec FA, Font RL. Orbit. In: Spencer WH, ed. Ophthalmic pathology: an atlas and textbook. Philadelphia: Saunders, 1986:2826–2831
53. Seidenberg KB, Lieb ML. Orbital myositis with Lyme disease. Am J Ophthalmol 1990;109:13–16
54. Donoso LA, Magargal LE, Eiferman RA. Fibrous dysplasia of the orbit with optic nerve decompression. Ann Ophthalmol 1982;14:80–83
55. Naiman J, Green WR, d'Heurle D, Iliff WJ. Brown tumor of the orbit associated with primary hyperparathyroidism. Am J Ophthalmol 1980;90:565–571
56. Ferry AP. Brown tumors (fibro-osseous bone replacement and overgrowth) of the orbit in hyperparathyroidism. Metab Pediatr Ophthalmol 1979;3:67–75
57. Whitson WE, Orcutt JC, Walkinshaw MD. Orbital osteoma in Gardner's syndrome. Am J Ophthalmol 1986;101:236–241
58. VanGehuchten DV, Lemagne J-M, Weber S. A case of exophthalmos—an early symptom of Gardner's syndrome. Orbit 1982;1:61–69
59. DeLaey JJ, DeSchryver A, Kluyskens P. Orbital involvement in Ollier's disease (multiple enchondromatosis). Int Ophthalmol 1982;5:149–154
60. Johnson TE, Nasr Am, Nalbandian RM, Cappelen-Smith J. Enchondromatosis and hemangioma (Maffucci's syndrome) with orbital involvement. Am J Ophthalmol 1990;110:153–159
61. Minton LR, Elliott JH. Ocular manifestations of infantile cortical hyperostosis. Am J Ophthalmol 1967;64:902–907
62. Morse PH, Walsh FB, McCormick JR. Ocular findings in hereditary diaphyseal dysplasia (Engelmann's disease). Am J Ophthalmol 1969;68:100–104
63. Beighton P, Hamersma H. Ophthalmological complications in the sclerosing bone dysplasias. Ophthalmol Pediatr Genet 1985;6(3):129–134
64. Bollersley J. Autosomal dominant osteopetrosis: bone metabolism, clinical and hormonal aspects. Endocr Rev 1989;10(1):45–67
65. Rathbun JE, Hoyt WF, Beard C. Surgical management of orbitofrontal varix in Klippel-Trenaunay-Weber syndrome. Am J Ophthalmol 1970;70:109–112
66. François J. Ocular aspects of the phakomatoses. In: Vinken PJ, Bruyn GW, eds. Handbook of clinical neurology. The phakomatoses, vol 14. New York: American Elsevier, 1972:619–663
67. Bloch RS, Gartner S. The incidence of ocular metastatic carcinoma. Arch Ophthalmol 1971;85:673–675
68. Shields CL, Shields JA, Peggs M. Metastatic tumors to the orbit. Ophthalmic Plast Reconstr Surg 1988;4:73–80
69. Rootman J. Diseases of the orbit. Philadelphia: Lippincott, 1988:405–427
70. Bertelsen TI. The premature synostosis of the cranial sutures. Acta Ophthalmol (Copenh) 1958;5(suppl):47–66
71. Nelson LB, Ingoglia S, Breinin GM. Sensorimotor disturbances in craniostenosis. J Pediatr Ophthalmol Strabismus 1981;18:32–41
72. Blank CE. Apert's syndrome (a type of acrocephalosyndactyly): observations in a British series of 39 cases. Ann Hum Genet 1960;24:151–173
73. Cohen MM. Cardiovascular anomalies in Apert's type acrocephalosyndactyly. Birth Defects 1982;8:239–241

Systemic Associations of Optic Neuritis

John A. McCrary, III, M.D.

Clinical Manifestations of Optic Neuritis

The purpose of this chapter is to outline succinctly the clinical presentation, examination and findings, many of the systemic associations, and laboratory assessment of optic neuritis. A few comments regarding diagnosis and treatment are included, but it is not possible here to detail all diagnostic findings, features, or treatment options for the diseases mentioned. Excellent references are available if details are desired.

It is imperative to distinguish optic neuritis from papilledema, which is caused by increased intracranial pressure but is not associated with a direct inflammatory reaction within the optic nerve or its dural sheath. A blurred distinction between optic neuritis and a number of optic neuropathies attributable to metabolic, degenerative, infiltrative, or vascular mechanisms has caused confusion. Any acquired, nonpapilledema optic nerve condition caused by a process without histopathological evidence of inflammation is best referred to as an optic neuropathy. This review is confined to those conditions that produce an inflammatory process within the optic nerve.

Clinical Onset

Optic neuritis is usually characterized as an acute, painful condition that produces rapid deterioration of vision in one or both eyes. In adult patients, uniocular disease is more common. In children, binocular onset of disease is not unusual. Occasional adults may present with bilateral, nearly simultaneous onset of optic neuritis. This unusual situation often suggests an acute neuropathic process such as Leber's optic neuropathy, particularly when it occurs in a male patient. The history of painful onset of disease, exaggerated by movement of the eyes, is atypical of optic neuropathy but is highly characteristic of an inflammatory process.

Most individuals with optic neuritis reach maximum loss of vision within the first 2 weeks after onset. Many patients note relative visual stabilization before 2 weeks is past. Continued downward spiraling of visual function beyond 2 weeks suggests another diagnosis. Optic neuritis victims often preserve good visual acuity even at the height of the disease. Yet the same individuals will display severe loss of visual field function and will complain of loss of light sense, disturbed color vision, and altered depth perception. Some patients will complain that attempted use of the impaired eye seems to hamper function in the normal fellow eye. Those so affected may close the eye or patch it in an attempt to minimize this complaint. Most optic neuritis patients quickly adapt and find patching unnecessary.

It is important to search the patient's past history for evidence of a possible causative factor for optic neuritis. Such a review should include questions regarding recent viral illnesses within 4 to 6 weeks before onset of optic neuritis. Risk factors for human immunodeficiency virus (HIV) infection should be assessed. Questions should be asked regarding weight loss, shortness of breath, cough, fever, or night sweats that might suggest sarcoidosis. Especially important are questions regarding previous neurological disease that might relate to the risk for multiple sclerosis. A history of myalgias, skin rash, fever, or joint pain could be compatible with collagen disease. Most patients who present with the first attack of optic neuritis are unaware of any of these conditions; they often have no pertinent history or complaints other than those pertaining to vision.

Visual Acuity Examination and Findings

The extent of visual acuity loss is highly variable. Some individuals will continue to maintain 20/15 to 20/40 visual acuity throughout the attack, whereas others will experience severe loss of visual acuity, even to no light perception [1, 2].

Visual Field Visual field defects found in individuals with optic neuritis show considerable variability. In the past, a central or cecocentral scotoma was believed to be most common. New evidence presented by Keltner [3] suggests 50% have generalized reduction of visual field function while the other half have focal defects. Among focal disorders of visual field, nearly 30% are altitudinal, 11% hemianopic, and only 8% cecocentral. Arcuate scotomas are even more unusual.

Pupils Examination of the pupil discloses significant loss of light sensitivity. The characteristic feature is the relative afferent pupil defect (Gunn pupil). This feature should be routinely detected when optic neuritis is present [4]. If this sign is not found, it suggests both eyes may have diminished sensory function or the cause for visual loss is not optic neuritis.

Contrast Sensitivity, Brightness, and Color Perception Defective contrast sensitivity is commonly encountered in acute optic neuritis. Individual complaints of loss of brightness sense and contrast sensitivity can be easily verified when clinical testing is performed [5]. Loss of brightness sense can be quantitated [6]. Loss of color vision is routinely encountered in optic neuritis. Color vision is often defective after optic neuritis recovery [7]. The most sensitive method for identifying such a color vision defect is the Farnsworth 100-

Hue test, though the use of pseudochromatic plates is usually more convenient and certainly less time-consuming. Even rapid comparison of color sense using red, green, or blue bottle tops from ophthalmic solution containers can confirm a difference in color perception of the affected eye as compared to its fellow. Color vision is often more severely affected than is visual acuity in individuals with acute optic neuritis.

Vitreous Examination of the vitreous may reveal a fine infiltrative hyalitis in individuals with optic neuritis. Heavy cellular infiltration suggests a serious underlying infectious or inflammatory condition causing optic neuritis. Such cases require more than routine evaluation and management. Conditions such as sarcoidosis or syphilitic optic neuritis are much more likely if this finding is present. The possibility of Lyme disease or HIV infection with its list of possible coinfections should be considered. Lymphoma may be seen presenting as visual loss presumed to be caused by optic neuritis combined with infiltrative vitreous reaction [8]. Cytological examination of vitreous aspirates and cerebrospinal fluid will provide the diagnosis quickly.

Fundus Ophthalmoscopic appearance of the optic nerve may be totally normal in retrobulbar optic neuritis. Although retrobulbar optic neuritis is the most common presentation, papillitis characterized by elevation of the optic nerve, hyperemia, vascular engorgement, and papillary or peripapillary splinter hemorrhages is not uncommon.

Combined inflammatory reaction in the optic nerve and retina—neuroretinitis—is characterized by papillitis with perifoveal exudates arranged in a starlike configuration.

■ Systemic Associations

Common Causes of Optic Neuritis

Although optic neuritis is often considered idiopathic, several common systemic associations are encountered. One should always be aware that underlying disease may be present or will manifest itself at some later date in an individual who presents with an isolated, first attack of optic neuritis. The most common disorder is multiple sclerosis; however, in today's medical environment the possibility of HIV-related diseases cannot be overlooked.

Multiple Sclerosis The common relationship of isolated optic neuritis with multiple sclerosis (MS) is widely known. No evidence has suggested that the clinical expression of optic neuritis associated with MS is any different from the idiopathic variety. The histopathology of disease appears to be no different when optic neuritis is created in experimental animals [9].

The risk of a relationship between MS and optic neuritis is considerably higher in patients between the ages of 20 and 40 years, particularly in women. This is especially true if length of follow-up is 5 years or longer. Within 5 years of onset of optic neuritis, more than 40% of women with isolated apparently idiopathic optic neuritis will manifest evidence of neurological disease compatible with a diagnosis of MS [10]. Longer follow-up appears to enhance the likelihood that MS will be diagnosed [11]. Magnetic resonance imaging (MRI) and spinal fluid examination done at initial presentation of optic neuritis often show findings compatible with the diagnosis. Earlier diagnosis may benefit patient management.

The philosophical debate regarding the need to inform the patient fully of the potential risk of MS remains unsettled. In most cases, patients appear to benefit by having the information of risk earlier. Such information may influence the patient to alter lifestyle by discontinuing the use of recreational drugs, smoking, abuse of alcohol, inappropriate dietary habits, and other anomalous patterns of behavior that may adversely affect immune function and thereby potentiate the risk for neurological disease. The recovery pattern of optic neuritis caused by MS appears no different from that of idiopathic origin. If optic neuritis recurs in the same eye, cumulative damage is the result: Visual function declines even more.

Postviral Optic Neuritis Postviral optic neuritis is a common condition most often encountered yearly from fall to spring. A significant number of adults and children will develop optic neuritis that appears to be related in some way to neurotrophic behavior of whatever virus is commonly found in the population at the time. The predominant virus causing widespread disease in a given population varies yearly. An exhaustive search for the underlying viral source is useless, but the history that the patient has had a recent viral contact within 4 to 6 weeks prior to the onset of disease is an important historical clue.

Many individuals with postviral optic neuritis may have forgotten about the viral attack until reminded. Some will develop optic nerve complications without a history of an upper respiratory infection, though members of the family may have had severe upper respiratory disease. The fact that a virus might clinically alter its presentation from an upper respiratory process to a neurological one within the same family group is recognized yet unexplained.

Neuroretinitis has a significant nonrelationship with MS; it is much more likely to be of viral or other postinfectious origin [12]. Neuroretinitis may rarely be caused by cat-scratch disease [13]. A history of a cat scratch followed by fever, malaise, lymphedema, and subsequent visual loss should prompt appropriate laboratory investigation and treatment.

Uncommon Causes of Optic Neuritis

HIV HIV-related diseases represent a more ominous group that may present with an attack of optic neuritis as the index manifestation of neurological disease. The patient may be totally unaware that he or she is HIV-positive. The patient may not recognize any of the potential risk factors. More and more heterosexual patients are becoming HIV-infected with no past history of drug abuse. The source is unprotected sexual activity.

Common conditions that may cause optic neuritis in a patient with HIV infection include syphilis, cytomegalovirus (CMV), herpes simplex, herpes zoster, toxoplasmosis, and cryptococcal fungal infection [14]. A patient may have any of these without HIV infection, but the risks of such diseases are higher if HIV infection coexists. The most common causes of HIV-related optic neuritis are syphilis [15] and CMV infection [16]. These are devastating central nervous system infections when encountered in HIV patients because the immunological compromise makes eradication of coinfectious disease difficult. The CMV patient will usually have typical CMV retinitis in conjunction with optic neuritis. Both CMV retinitis and herpes simplex retinitis cause sheetlike necrosis of retina with intense vasculitis, occlusion of arterioles, and subsequent necrosis. Untreated, these are relentlessly progressive. Cryptococcal retinitis appears as a fluffy infiltration of choroid and retina. Sheetlike necrosis is not a feature. Hyalitis is usually seen over the area of involvement, much as with toxoplasmosis. Optic neuritis may be a feature of cryptococcal infection associated with cryptococcal arachnoiditis in acquired immunodeficiency syndrome (AIDS) patients [17].

If a patient is HIV-positive, a computed tomography or MRI scan, spinal fluid examination, and complete evaluation of the serological and spinal fluid markers for CMV, syphilis, and cryptococcal disease should be obtained. Vitreous samples may be needed to confirm the diagnosis in some patients. Appropriate management is targeted on the HIV-associated disease or diseases identified clinically and by laboratory assessment as the cause of vision loss.

Sarcoidosis Sarcoidosis is frequently overlooked as a cause of optic neuritis [18]. It is often encountered in patients 20 to 40 years of age. Black and white patients of Northern European ancestry are most often afflicted. Such patients receive an incorrect diagnosis of idiopathic optic neuritis that fails to respond adequately to steroid therapy or immediately reactivates when treatment is stopped. Failure to obtain a routine chest roentgenogram before initiating treatment with oral corticosteroids is usually the explanation for failure to diagnose sarcoidosis.

Some individuals with sarcoidosis will present with elevated sedimentation rate, facial rash, and lymphadenopathy that could be misinterpreted as a viral illness or connective tissue disease such as systemic lupus erythematosus. The identification of an elevated sedimentation rate but normal antinuclear antibody (ANA) in a patient with a lupuslike facial rash should raise the possibility of sarcoidosis. A few patients will have central nervous system sarcoidosis yet fail to manifest typical mediastinal infiltration on routine chest roentgenography. Extrapulmonary sarcoidosis without any evidence of hilar lymphadenopathy is rare.

Evaluation of angiotensin-converting enzyme (ACE) serum levels, gallium scans of the lacrimal glands, and conjunctival biopsy are all adjunctive diagnostic methods. Conjunctival biopsy is least valuable; elevated ACE levels are present in 60 to 80% of patients with active sarcoidosis. Biopsy confirmation of enlarged lymph nodes is absolutely diagnostic.

Connective Tissue Disease Connective tissue diseases, among which lupus is the leading concern, may present as isolated optic neuritis. This autoimmune optic neuritis must be recognized early since adequate steroid therapy appears to be critical to proper management [19].

Autoimmune disease may not be readily apparent by clinical history or physical examination. Laboratory studies for elevated ANA, antinative DNA, sedimentation rate, or other serological markers of connective tissue disease are important. These patients need treatment with corticosteroids [20, 21]. Treatment may have to be continued for a very long time; therefore, these patients must be identified early. A rheumatologist should be consulted.

Non-HIV Viral Diseases Specific viral illnesses unassociated with HIV, such as mumps [22] and measles [23], have been reported to produce optic neuritis. However, these are rarely encountered in routine practice. Clinical features of either condition should make the diagnosis. The onset of unilateral or bilateral optic neuritis may be encountered. Clinical manifestations of optic neuritis appear to be no different from those found with other non-HIV viral illnesses. Optic neuritis may also follow chickenpox [24] (varicella-zoster virus) in childhood or adult life.

Nonsyphilitic Bacterial Diseases Less common bacterial diseases that can cause optic neuritis include tuberculosis [25] and Lyme disease [26], caused by the treponeme *Borrelia bergdorferi*. Serological testing for Lyme disease is usually diagnostic. Lyme disease is especially likely if the patient has a prior history of migratory, erythematous skin rash (erythema multiforme migrans) and arthralgias together with optic neuritis or uveitis. Lyme disease can cause many different clinical expressions of ocular disease, much the same as syphilis. Antibiotic treatment is curative.

Parasitic Diseases Parasitic diseases that may cause optic neuritis are toxoplasmosis [27] and infection with *Toxocara canis* [28]. Toxoplasmosis, which may or may not be associated with HIV infection, causes an intense retinochoroiditis with secondary hyalitis. Optic neuritis can be a feature of active inflammatory disease caused by toxoplasmosis. The clinical findings are usually an old, retinochoroidal, dense white scar in the posterior pole with nearby active whitish to yellowish, fluffy retinitis. The vitreous reaction may be sufficiently intense that the fundus cannot be well seen. If toxoplasmosis is suspected, corticosteroids should never be used until specific treatment for the infection has begun.

The *Toxocara* organism may directly invade through the optic nerves, subsequently gain access to the intraocular compartment, and then proceed through the vitreous cavity anteriorly to generate the typical endovitreal opacity that points to a peripheral retinal scar. Serological diagnostic tests and specific treatments are available for each of these disorders.

Fungal Diseases Fungal illnesses that may cause optic neuritis or combined retinal and optic nerve inflammatory reaction in patients without AIDS include aspergillosis [29], cryptococcosis [30], and histoplasmosis [31] (rare). When ocular histoplasmosis causes optic neuritis, typical chorioretinal and peripapillary scars are present. The lesions do not contain active organisms but are of probable immune origin. Reactivation of peripapillary disease can cause secondary optic neuritis. Steroid treatment of the inflammatory reaction is usually very effective. Occasionally, photocoagulation is required. Aspergillosis, cryptococcosis, and other deep fungal infections, on the other hand, are treated with amphotericin B or other antifungal agents.

Steroids should never be given to a patient with active deep fungal infection until antifungal therapy is started. Even then, extreme caution is required. Aspergillosis presenting as a steroid-sensitive optic neuritis has been reported. Complications caused by steroid therapy invariably occur when treatment is given before adequate evaluation is carried out and antifungal therapy is started.

Unusual Retinal Diseases Unusual diseases with which optic neuritis may be associated include diffuse unilateral subacute neuroretinitis (DUSN) [32], acute retinal necrosis (ARN) [33], acute posterior multifocal placoid pigment epitheliopathy (APMPPE), and multiple evanescent white dot syndrome (MEWDS). Each of these appears as a diffuse retinopathy or pigment epithelial disorder. Neuritis is a secondary process. If the cerebrospinal fluid does not show evidence of an inflammatory process and the optic nerve does not have diffuse late staining on fluorescein angiography, vision loss is more likely due to retinopathy alone.

DUSN is of parasitic origin [32]. The organism is probably the larval form of *Bayliascaris procyonis.* Laser photocoagulation can destroy the organism. Release of toxic byproducts from death of the larva can cause intense inflammation that requires treatment with corticosteroids.

ARN is caused by herpesvirus infection [33]. Treatment with intravenous acyclovir is most effective. Both APMPPE and MEWDS are of uncertain cause but may follow a viral prodrome and tend to be self-limited [34–36]. No specific treatment exists for either. Corticosteroids may be useful. Optic neuritis may be found with birdshot retinochoroidopathy [37].

Rare Diseases Other rare conditions of unknown cause with which optic neuritis may be associated are Behçet's disease [38] and Devic's disease. Behçet's disease classically presents in individuals of Middle Eastern or Mediterranean descent but may be found worldwide and causes chronic uveitis, aphthous ulcers of the mouth and genitalia, and cutaneous lesions. Prevalent central nervous system manifestations include optic neuritis, seizures, and encephalopathy. Behçet's disease is best treated with combinations of corticosteroids and cyclophosphamide or chlorambucil. The disease shares many of the features of Reiter's syndrome.

Devic's disease (neuromyelitis optica) has two key features: bilateral optic neuritis and ascending transverse myelitis. The condition may be a form of MS, but some patients develop the condition after a viral illness [39]. Treatment usually is high-dose corticosteroids and supportive management, much as with Guillain-Barré syndrome, in which optic neuritis also may be a feature.

Postvaccination optic neuritis [40], inflammatory bowel disease [41], Wegener's granulomatosis [42], and severe, pyogenic sinus infection [43] are among those rare conditions that may occasionally cause optic neuritis.

■ Laboratory Assessment

The minimum required laboratory assessment of a patient with optic neuritis must include the following studies: (1) chest roentgenogram, (2) ANA titer, (3) sedimentation rate, (4) microhemagglutination-treponema pallidum

(MHA-TP) or fluorescent treponemal antibody absorption (FTA-Abs) test with rapid plasma reagin (RPR), (5) HIV testing (with patient's permission), and (6) fasting blood sugar (FBS). An FBS should be obtained before steroid treatment to rule out occult diabetes mellitus. A urine pregnancy test should be done on all women of child-bearing age. All of these should be reviewed *before* the patient is treated with corticosteroids, if steroid treatment is planned.

If the practitioner is concerned about the possibility that MS may be a contributing factor, an MRI scan of brain and orbits should be obtained. Special attention should be focused on the optic nerves. Fat suppression sequences may be helpful as the optic nerve anatomy can be better displayed by this method. Gadolinium enhancement is advocated to assist in excluding possible concerns of optic nerve tumor or intracranial tumor. Such concerns are justified particularly when progression of visual loss continues beyond 2 to 3 weeks, other cranial nerves are affected, or a history of progressive weight loss, severe headaches, or altered mentation is detected.

A complete neurological examination should be performed if MS is suspected or the history suggests the need. The question of a lumbar puncture is often raised. Most patients do not want a lumbar puncture, but the diagnostic advantage of spinal fluid assessment combined with MRI can aid in answering questions about MS, central nervous system infection, or neoplastic processes [44]. Spinal fluid testing is not needed for most routine optic neuritis patients who have had only one attack. Those with more than one attack or other new neurological symptoms should have a spinal tap.

A much larger array of diagnostic tests is required to rule out less common causes of optic neuritis when clinically indicated.

■ Treatment

A detailed review of all treatment options for each disease described here is beyond the scope or intent of this chapter. Some of these have already been mentioned briefly as each disease was discussed. An excellent resource that details the laboratory workup, diagnosis, and treatment of each of these conditions is recommended [45].

If no disease that requires specialized treatment is identified, many ophthalmologists are content to observe the patient until the customary recovery phase of optic neuritis begins within a few weeks after the onset of the condition. The best visual outcome usually occurs within the first 3 to 6 months after the onset of the process but may occur much more rapidly. Approximately 70% of patients will have what is considered a good outcome (20/40 or better) after one attack of optic neuritis.

Some studies suggest that patients who are observed, as a group, have essentially the same visual outcome as those who are treated with potent corticosteroids. Other studies indicate steroid treatment provides the patient with an enhanced outcome. Routes of treatment vary. Oral high-dose, intravenous megadose, and retrobulbar repository administration of steroids have received support. No common agreement exists with respect to route of administration, timing, dose, or choice of medication. Therefore, the whole issue of steroid therapy for optic neuritis remains unsettled. For this reason, the Optic Neuritis

Treatment Trial, which began in 1987, has been enrolling patients nationwide to be randomized in a controlled, prospective study designed to determine the actual benefit of corticosteroid therapy in treating optic neuritis [46]. The enrollment phase of the study will be concluded in June 1991. Publication of data will be forthcoming within a few months of concluding enrollment. This study should conclusively answer questions regarding the benefit or nonbenefit of steroid therapy in individuals with optic neuritis and, at the same time, will provide an enormous body of data regarding the risks for MS in this population.

■ Conclusion

The primary job of the ophthalmologist who encounters a patient with the first attack of optic neuritis is to rule out likely cofactors for disease. If a treatable etiological agent can be identified by history and laboratory testing, specific therapy should be given. Optic neuritis may be the first manifestation of a disease that is systemic and dangerous if left untreated. Failure to subject the patient to a reasonable number of diagnostic studies represents a serious oversight and should be avoided. Only a few laboratory studies need be obtained in most patients with optic neuritis. If these studies are unremarkable, one then has to decide whether to treat with corticosteroids or observe the patient.

Patients who do not follow the typical behavior pattern for optic neuritis certainly deserve a much more aggressive evaluation in the laboratory. Slowly progressive loss of vision is inconsistent with optic neuritis. The description *chronic optic neuritis* is to be avoided, since most patients who have progression of visual loss beyond 2 to 3 weeks are much more likely to have a neoplasm or other very serious problem as its cause. Chronic optic neuritis is best abandoned as a useful diagnosis.

The indiscriminate use of steroids in managing patients with optic neuritis without access to an adequate number of laboratory studies is a common failure in practice and should be avoided. If the physician does not wish to perform any laboratory studies on the patient, it is probably wise to withhold steroid therapy.

■ References

1. Miller NR. Walsh and Hoyt's clinical neuro-ophthalmology, ed 4, vol 1. Baltimore: Williams & Wilkins, 1982:227–248
2. Perkin GD, Rose FC. Optic neuritis and its differential diagnosis. Oxford: Oxford Medical, 1979
3. Keltner JL, Johnson CA, Spurr JO. Optic neuritis treatment trial (ONTT): initial visual field defects (poster presentation). Atlanta, GA: American Academy of Ophthalmology, 1990
4. Cox TA, Thompson SH, Corbett JJ. Relative afferent pupil defects in optic neuritis. Am J Ophthalmol 1981;92:685–690
5. Beck RW, Ruchman MC, Savino PJ, et al. Contrast sensitivity measurements in acute and resolved optic neuritis. Br J Ophthalmol 1984;68:756–759

6. Sadun AA, Lessell S. Brightness-sense and optic nerve disease. Arch Ophthalmol 1985;103:39–43
7. Fleishman JA, Beck RW, Linares OA, et al. Deficits in visual function after resolution of optic neuritis. Ophthalmology 1987;94:1029–1035
8. Kattah JC, Suski ET, Killen JY, et al. Optic neuritis and systemic lymphoma. Am J Ophthalmol 1980;89:431–436
9. Sergott RC, Brown MJ, Polenta RMD, et al. Optic nerve demyelination induced by human serum: patients with multiple sclerosis or optic neuritis and normal subjects. Neurology (NY) 1985;35:1438–1442
10. Cohen MM, Lessell S, Wolf PA. A prospective study of the risk of developing multiple sclerosis in uncomplicated optic neuritis. Neurology (NY) 1979;29:208–213
11. Rizzo JF, Lessell S: Risk of developing multiple sclerosis after uncomplicated optic neuritis: A long-term prospective study. Neurology (NY) 1988;38:185–190
12. Dreyer RF, Hopen G, Gass JD, et al. Leber's idiopathic stellate neuroretinitis. Arch Ophthalmol 1984;102:1140–1145
13. Chrousos GA, Drack AV, Young M, et al. Neuroretinitis in cat-scratch disease. J Clin Neuro Ophthalmol 1990;10:92–94
14. Mansour AM. Neuro-ophthalmic findings in acquired immunodeficiency syndrome. J Clin Neuro Ophthalmol 1990;10:167–174
15. Carter JB, Hamill RJ, Matoba AY. Bilateral syphilitic optic neuritis in a patient with a positive test for HIV. Arch Ophthalmol 1987;105:1485–1486
16. Grossniklaus HE, Frank KE, Tomsak RL. Cytomegalovirus retinitis and optic neuritis in acquired immunodeficiency syndrome: report of a case. Ophthalmology 1987;94:1601–1604
17. Lipson BK, Freeman WR, Beniz J, et al. Optic neuropathy associated with cryptococcal arachnoiditis in AIDS patients. Am J Ophthalmol 1989;107:523–527
18. Galetta S, Shatz NJ, Glaser JS. Acute sarcoid optic neuropathy with spontaneous recovery. J Clin Neuro Ophthalmol 1989;9:27–32
19. Kupersmith MJ, Burde RM, Warren FA, et al. Autoimmune optic neuropathy: evaluation and treatment. J Neurol Neurosurg Psychiatry 1988;51:1381–1386
20. Kimberly RP, Lockshin MD, Sherman RL, et al. High-dose intravenous methylprednisolone pulse therapy in systemic lupus erythematosus patients. Am J Med 1981;70:817–824
21. Spoor TC. Treatment of optic neuritis with megadose corticosteroids. J Clin Neuro Ophthalmol 1986;6:137–143
22. Foster RE, Lowder CY, Meisler DM, et al. Mumps neuroretinitis in an adolescent. Am J Ophthalmol 1990;110:91–93
23. Connolly JH, Hutchinson WM, Allen IV, et al. Carotid artery thrombosis, encephalitis, myelitis and optic neuritis associated with rubella virus infections. Brain 1975;98:583–594
24. Purvin V, Hrisomalos N, Dunn D. Varicella optic neuritis. Neurology (NY) 1988;38:501–503
25. Fruchtman SM, Banerji MA. Tuberculous meningitis: diagnostic problem of visual loss and diabetes insipidus during treatment. NY State J Med 1980;80:963–965
26. Winward KE, Smith JL, Culbertson WW, et al. Ocular Lyme borreliosis. Am J Ophthalmol 1989;108:651–657
27. Roach ES, Zimmerman CF, Troost BT, et al. Optic neuritis due to acquired toxoplasmosis. Pediatr Neurol 1985;1:114–116
28. Margo CE, Sedwick LA, Rubin ML. Neuroretinitis in presumed visceral larva migrans. Retina 1986;6:95–98
29. Spoor TC, Hartel WC, Harding S, et al. Aspergillosis presenting as a corticosteroid responsive optic neuropathy. J Clin Neuro Ophthalmol 1982;2:103–107

30. Kupfer C, McCrane E. A possible cause of decreased vision in cryptococcal meningitis. Invest Ophthalmol 1974;13:801–804
31. Husted RC, Shock JP. Acute presumed histoplasmosis of the optic nerve head. Br J Ophthalmol 1975;59:409–412
32. Kazacos KR, Raymond LA, Kazacos EA, et al. The raccoon ascarid. A probable cause of human ocular larva migrans. Ophthalmology 1985;92:1735–1744
33. Sergott RC, Belmont JB, Savino PJ, et al. Optic nerve involvement in the acute retinal necrosis syndrome. Arch Ophthalmol 1985;103:1160–1162
34. Folk JC, Pulido JS, Wolf MD. White dot chorioretinal inflammatory syndromes. San Francisco: American Academy of Ophthalmology (clinical module), 1990;8(2):1–10
35. Aaberg TM. Multiple evanescent white dot syndrome [letter]. Arch Ophthalmol 1988;106:1162–1163
36. Kirkham TH, Ffytche TJ, Sanders MD. Placoid pigment epitheliopathy with retinal vasculitis and papillitis. Br J Ophthalmol 1972;56:875–880
37. Soubrane G, Bokobza R, Coscas G. Late developing lesions in birdshot retinochoroidopathy. Am J Ophthalmol 1990;109:204–210
38. Kansu T, Kirkali P, Kansu E, et al. Optic neuropathy in Behçet's disease. J Clin Neuro Ophthalmol 1989;9:277–280
39. Chusid MJ, Williamson SJ, Murphy JV, et al. Neuromyelitis optica (Devic disease) following varicella infection. J Pediatr 1979;95:737–738
40. Kline LB, Margulies SL, Oh SJ. Optic neuritis and myelitis following rubella vaccination. Arch Neurol 1982;39:443–444
41. Macoul KL. Ocular changes in granulomatous ileocolitis. Arch Ophthalmol 1970;84:95–97
42. Haynes BF, Fishman ML, Frauci AS, et al. The ocular manifestations of Wegener's granulomatosis. Fifteen years' experience and a review of the literature. Am J Med 1977;63:131–141
43. Awerbuch G, Labadie EL, Van Dalen JT. Reversible optic neuritis secondary to paranasal sinusitis. Eur Neurol 1989;29:189–193
44. Miller JR, Burke AM, Bever CT. Occurrence of oligoclonal bands in multiple sclerosis and other CNS diseases. Ann Neurol 1983;13:53–58
45. Fraunfelder FT, Roy FH. Current ocular therapy, 3rd edition. Philadelphia: Saunders, 1990
46. Beck RW. The Optic Neuritis Treatment Trial [Editorial]. Arch Ophthalmol 1988;106:1051–1053

Index

Future Issues

Volume 31, 1991

Fall (No. 4)

NEURO-OPHTHALMOLOGY
Lanning B. Kline, M.D., Guest Editor

Volume 32, 1992

Winter (No. 1)

PEDIATRIC OPHTHALMOLOGY
Frederick A. Jakobiec, M.D., and Dimitri Azar, M.D., Guest Editors

Spring (No. 2)

RETINAL AND VITREAL SURGERY
Joseph Olk, M.D., Guest Editor

Summer (No. 3)

ORBITAL DISEASE
John Shore, M.D., Guest Editor

Fall (No. 4)

COMPLICATIONS IN OPHTHALMIC SURGERY